Fast Facts for the CATH LAB NURSE (*McCulloch*)

Fast Facts About NEUROCRITICAL CARE: A Quick Reference for the Advanced Practice Provider (*McLaughlin*)

Fast Facts for DEMENTIA CARE: What Nurses Need to Know in a Nutshell (*Miller*)

Fast Facts for HEALTH PROMOTION IN NURSING: Promoting Wellness in a Nutshell (*Miller*)

Fast Facts for STROKE CARE NURSING: An Expert Care Guide, Second Edition (*Morrison*)

Fast Facts for the MEDICAL OFFICE NURSE: What You Really Need to Know in a Nutshell (*Richmeier*)

Fast Facts for the PEDIATRIC NURSE: An Orientation Guide in a Nutshell (*Rupert, Young*)

Fast Facts About FORENSIC NURSING: What You Need to Know (*Scannell*)

Fast Facts About the GYNECOLOGICAL EXAM: A Professional Guide for NPs, PAs, and Midwives, Second Edition (*Secor, Fantasia*)

Fast Facts for the STUDENT NURSE: Nursing Student Success in a Nutshell (*Stabler-Haas*)

Fast Facts About RELIGION FOR NURSES: Implications for Patient Care (*Taylor*)

Fast Facts for CAREER SUCCESS IN NURSING: Making the Most of Mentoring in a Nutshell (*Vance*)

Fast Facts for the TRIAGE NURSE: An Orientation and Care Guide, Second Edition (*Visser, Montejano*)

Fast Facts for DEVELOPING A NURSING ACADEMIC PORTFOLIO: What You Really Need to Know in a Nutshell (*Wittmann-Price*)

Fast Facts for the HOSPICE NURSE: A Concise Guide to End-of-Life Care (*Wright*)

Fast Facts for the CLASSROOM NURSING INSTRUCTOR: Classroom Teaching in a Nutshell (*Yoder-Wise, Kowalski*)

Forthcoming FAST FACTS Books

Fast Facts for NURSE PRACTITIONERS: Current Practice Essentials for the Clinical Subspecialties (*Atkan*)

Fast Facts for the ER NURSE: Guide to a Successful Emergency Department Orientation, Fourth Edition (*Buettner*)

Fast Facts for WRITING THE DNP PROJECT: Effective Structure, Content, and Presentation (*Christenbery*)

Fast Facts for the NURSE PRECEPTOR: Keys to Providing a Successful Preceptorship, Second Edition (*Ciocco*)

Fast Facts for the NEONATAL NURSE: Care Essentials for Normal and High-Risk Neonates, Second Edition (*Davidson*)

Fast Facts About NEUROPATHIC PAIN: What Advanced Practice Nurses and Physician Assistants Need to Know (*Davies*)

Fast Facts about DIVERSITY, EQUITY, AND INCLUSION (*Davis*)

Fast Facts for CREATING A SUCCESSFUL TELEHEALTH SERVICE: A How-to Guide for Nurse Practitioners (*Heidesch*)

Fact Facts for NURSE ANESTHESIA (*Hickman*)

Fast Facts for PATIENT SAFETY IN NURSING (*Hunt*)

Fast Facts for DEMENTIA CARE: What Nurses Need to Know, Second Edition (*Miller*)

Fast Facts for DNP ROLE DEVELOPMENT: A Career Navigation Guide (*Menonna-Quinn, Tortorella Genova*)

Fast Facts for MAKING THE MOST OF YOUR CAREER IN NURSING (*Redulla*)

Fast Facts for PEDIATRIC PRIMARY CARE: A Guide for Nurse Practitioners and Physician Assistants (*Ruggiero*)

Fast Facts About SEXUALLY TRANSMITTED INFECTIONS (STIs): A Nurse's Guide to Expert Patient Care (*Scannell*)

Fast Facts for the CLINICAL NURSE LEADER (*Wilcox, Deerhake*)

Fast Facts for the HOSPICE NURSE: A Concise Guide to End-of-Life Care, Second Edition (*Wright*)

FAST FACTS for
THE CRITICAL CARE NURSE

Dina Hewett, PhD, RN, CCRN, NEA-BC, received her BSN from Brenau University, MSN from Georgia Southern University, and PhD in higher education from the University of Georgia. Her certifications include Critical Care Registered Nurse (Alumnus) and Nurse Executive Advanced. She is also certified as a Six Sigma Black Belt. Dr. Hewett has over 30 years of experience as a critical care nurse, and her career has encompassed both hospital administration and academics. During her tenure in hospital administration, she served as the unit manager of the cardiothoracic ICU and director of nursing of multiple units, including critical care, inpatient rehabilitation, and respiratory therapy.

Dr. Hewett is an AACN-Wharton Executive Fellow, a treasurer of the Georgia Nurses Association, a board member of the Georgia Association of Nursing Deans and Directors, and a member of the Education Committee of the Georgia Board of Nursing.

FAST FACTS for
THE CRITICAL CARE NURSE

Second Edition

Dina Hewett, PhD, RN, CCRN, NEA-BC

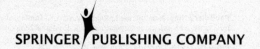

SPRINGER PUBLISHING COMPANY

Springer Publishing Company, LLC
11 West 42nd Street
New York, NY 10036
www.springerpub.com
http://connect.springerpub.com

Acquisitions Editor: Rachel Landes
Compositor: Amnet Systems

ISBN: 978-0-8261-7716-2
ebook ISBN: 978-0-8261-7721-6
DOI: 10.1891/9780826177216

20 21 22 / 5 4 3

The author and the publisher of this work have made every effort to use sources believed to be reliable to provide information that is accurate and compatible with the standards generally accepted at the time of publication. Because medical science is continually advancing, our knowledge base continues to expand. Therefore, as new information becomes available, changes in procedures become necessary. We recommend that the reader always consult current research and specific institutional policies before performing any clinical procedure. The author and publisher shall not be liable for any special, consequential, or exemplary damages resulting, in whole or in part, from the readers' use of, or reliance on, the information contained in this book. The publisher has no responsibility for the persistence or accuracy of URLs for external or third-party Internet websites referred to in this publication and does not guarantee that any content on such websites is, or will remain, accurate or appropriate.

Library of Congress Cataloging-in-Publication Data

Names: Hewett, Dina, author. | Landrum, Michele Angell. Fast facts for the critical care nurse.
Title: Fast facts for the critical care nurse / Dina Hewett.
Other titles: Fast facts (Springer Publishing Company)
Description: Second edition. | New York, NY : Springer Publishing Company, LLC, [2020] | Series: Fast facts | Preceded by Fast facts for the critical care nurse / Michele Angell Landrum. c2012. | Includes bibliographical references and index.
Identifiers: LCCN 2019035724 (print) | LCCN 2019035725 (ebook) | ISBN 9780826177162 (paperback) | ISBN 9780826177216 (ebook)
Subjects: MESH: Critical Illness—nursing | Critical Care—methods | Critical Care Nursing
Classification: LCC RC86.7 (print) | LCC RC86.7 (ebook) | NLM WY 154 | DDC 616.02/8—dc23
LC record available at https://lccn.loc.gov/2019035724
LC ebook record available at https://lccn.loc.gov/2019035725

Publisher's Note: New and used products purchased from third-party sellers are not guaranteed for quality, authenticity, or access to any included digital components.

Printed in the United States of America.

Contents

Contents

Part III PATIENT- AND FAMILY-CENTERED CARE

Preface

I remember that, as a graduate nurse beginning my career in critical care, the learning curve was steep! In those days, I continuously read books and journals and attended as many continuing education events as possible. I needed a reference manual that provided a quick, concise review of the most common diagnoses and interventions. I have attempted to compile that type of reference in this book.

Designed for a new or recent graduate transitioning into the critical care environment, this book provides a quick reference of the most common admitting diagnoses in critical care, including causes, signs and symptoms, and interventions, that will be used every day. Part I reviews the foundational aspects of critical care nursing, including the critical care environment, the electronic medical record, and specialty certifications for the critical care nurse. Obtaining certification in critical care nursing signifies commitment, professionalism, and continuing education in critical care. Chapter 4 is dedicated to an area that is often overlooked or ignored . . . self-care. Taking care of yourself as a critical care nurse is just as vital as taking care of your patients. Self-care will help you maintain your health when working in a highly stressful and complex environment.

Part II covers critical care nursing in a systemic approach. Starting with neurological care in Chapter 5 and proceeding through each body system, the chapters begin with an assessment and then provide the most common admitting diagnoses. Each diagnosis is presented with a cause, signs and symptoms, and interventions. Each chapter discusses the critical aspects of caring for a patient presenting with a specific diagnosis. Chapter 6 provides an overview of supplemental oxygenation methods and ventilator functions and settings in addition to common disease states. Chapter 7 provides an overview of the care of patients with heart disease along with information on cardiovascular support devices: intra-aortic balloon pump, temporary pacing, ventricular assist devices, and the Impella device. Chapter 8 provides an overview of the different types of shock states with a focus on septic shock and the updated bundled-care approach for treating patients presenting with sepsis and septic shock. Chapter 9 encompasses upper and lower GI bleeding, acute pancreatitis, and hepatic encephalopathy. Chapter 10 includes an overview of acute kidney injury and specific interventions for patient support such as continuous renal replacement therapy. Chapter 11 includes an overview of the common endocrine-related critical care disease states, including diabetic ketoacidosis and hyperosmolar hyperglycemic state. Chapter 12 provides an overview of blunt and penetrating trauma leading to injury of the brain, thorax, abdomen, and musculoskeletal system. Chapter 13 reviews patient care for the most common transplant procedures. The care of the burn patient is discussed in Chapter 14, including burn classification, severity, and general care guidelines.

Part III focuses on patient- and family-centered care at the end of life. Chapter 15 provides guidelines for withdrawal of treatment, palliative care, and the generalized protocol for a terminal wean that can help facilitate a "good" death. Chapter 16 provides a comparison of palliative care and hospice care. Further, the palliative care bundle is presented as a care approach in the critical care environment. Finally, Chapter 17 provides an overview of the care of the organ donor patient.

The new graduate nurse beginning a career or the experienced nurse transitioning to critical care should never stop yearning for new knowledge and should take advantage of every opportunity to expand your knowledge base—always ask questions, develop a strong network, and identify a mentor to guide you along the way. You have to develop a thick skin, but never lose your compassion and empathy. Always advocate for your patient because at the end of the shift, the patient is what matters the most!

Dina Hewett

Acknowledgments

In my career as a critical care nurse, I have had the honor and privilege of learning from the best. From my first experience in critical care as a new graduate in a well-structured residency-type program to the start-up of a cardiothoracic program, my professional life has been enriched by mentors and teachers. Now as an educator, my goal is to mentor and educate the next critical care nurse to provide excellent patient care.

For my nursing students who inspire me with their dedication and commitment to the nursing profession: Never stop learning. Healthcare is a dynamic profession that will require you to learn every day. You have the honor and privilege of interacting with patients and families during the most joyous and saddest moments in their lives. Never lose sight of that honor.

This book would not be possible without the love and support of my family: My mom Gloria's unconditional love and support; my son, Lincoln, who made me a mom; and my husband Chuck's who gave me unwavering love and support while I worked on this book every weekend.

I

Foundational Issues in Critical Care Nursing

1

The Critical Care Environment

The American Association of Critical-Care Nurses (AACN) defines critical care nursing as "a specialty within nursing that deals specifically with human responses to life-threatening problems" (2010, April). Critical care units range from open heart recovery units, burn units, and neurological ICUs to surgical ICUs, medical ICUs, and cardiac care units. All have distinct qualities while sharing several similar attributes.

Nurses who thrive in these areas are highly specialized and educated to assess patients efficiently and to provide appropriate, proficient, culturally relevant, and emotionally sensitive care for both the patient and the family. These are the core values of critical care nursing.

Critical care nurses maintain the highest quality of care for patients, work collaboratively in an interdisciplinary team, and are an advocate for their patients and families.

In this chapter, you will learn:

1. The qualifications for critical care nurses
2. The different types of critical care units
3. The standards and scope of care identified by the AACN

QUALIFICATIONS

Most nurses who are interested in a critical care position already possess the appropriate requirements. These include:

1. An active, unencumbered registered nursing license in the state of employment
2. Current Basic Life Support (BLS)
3. Current Advanced Cardiac Life Support (ACLS)

A critical care nurse must be able to carefully assess patients with complex health conditions, plan care to meet their needs, implement the care, and evaluate the interventions. All this must be done simultaneously, consistently, and rapidly.

Critical care nurses share many traits with others practicing throughout the nursing spectrum. They are organized, ethical, proficient, caring, humane, respectful, eager to learn, cool under pressure, and confident. Nurses always keep what is best for the patient foremost, thereby ensuring that proper care is given. Once hired, a critical care nurse completes hospital and unit orientations. A nurse is assigned a preceptor to facilitate unit orientation. Education and training must be ongoing throughout critical care nursing to ensure up-to-date skills and competency.

Many hospitals now offer nurse residency programs in critical care. These programs provide a structured orientation process with continuing education. Generally designed for a new graduate nurse, these residency programs may last between 12 and 18 weeks, combining classroom education with precepted patient care in the critical care unit. The new nurse is mentored and guided throughout the residency with frequent opportunities for feedback, evaluation, and education. Depending on the size and complexity of the organization, rotation through the different types of critical care units may be part of the residency program. During the residency, the new nurse may complete ACLS certification.

TYPES OF CRITICAL CARE UNITS

There are a variety of settings and types of critical care units, including coronary, medical, and surgical ICUs, as well as highly specialized units such as cardiovascular/thoracic, transplant, and burn units. TeleICU is now a specialized care provided by critical care nurses in remote locations, utilizing closed-circuit monitoring for assessment and evaluation. Through this technology, nurses can consult with highly trained healthcare providers.

Although all critical care units have similarities, several items and situations vary according to the particular type of critical care area. The number of patient beds or rooms is generally the biggest variant.

A unit may have 2 beds or 25 to 30 beds, depending on the hospital size, location, and specialty demand.

Fast Facts

Common Characteristics of Critical Care Units

1. A nurse-to-patient ratio of 1:1 or 1:2
2. Critically ill patients
3. Patients with multiple diagnoses and comorbidities
4. Continuous monitoring: EKG, blood pressure, oxygen saturation, respiratory rate
5. Specialized equipment: Multiple IV pumps, chest tubes, ventilators, intra-aortic balloon pump (IABP), continuous renal replacement therapy (CRRT), extracorporeal membrane oxygenation (ECMO), and left ventricular assist device (LVAD)
6. Invasive monitoring: Arterial line, pulmonary artery catheter, central venous pressure, intracranial pressure (ICP), and ventriculostomy
7. Isolation precautions
8. Bedside computers for documentation and access to patient information

The type of patients in intensive care varies according to the facility, unit type, and staff and bed availability. Usually, a facility has a general ICU that is a catchall for most patients and a surgical ICU for postsurgical patients. Both units utilize most of the equipment mentioned earlier, as well as other items, such as a IABP and continuous venovenous hemodialysis (CVVHD) machine. Other types of critical care units include:

- The *surgical intensive care unit* (SICU) is where patients recover after highly complex invasive surgery, such as a Whipple procedure, orthopedic reconstruction, or complex abdominal repair. They often have additional medical conditions that require close monitoring and special treatment.
- Patients in the *neurological intensive care unit* (neuro-ICU) require detailed care pertaining to their neurological status. They might have experienced a stroke, may exhibit increased ICP, have suffered acute head trauma, or may be comatose. An ICP monitor

and/or drain may be inserted and maintained in this patient care setting.

- The *cardiac care unit* (CCU) is common in most hospitals and is used for patients experiencing some type of cardiac issue, including unstable angina, myocardial infarction (MI), post-stent placement for an ST-elevated MI, or postcardiothoracic surgery for a coronary artery bypass. An IABP is often used in the CCU.

- The *cardiovascular intensive care unit* (CVICU) is generally for postcardiac bypass patients. However, other patients may be admitted to this unit, including those with postoperative thoracic aneurysm repair, abdominal aneurysm repair, and thoracotomies. IABPs, LVADs, biventricular assist devices (BIVADs), and CVVHD devices are often used in this unit.

- Nurses in the *transplant unit*, where post–organ transplant patients recover, are trained specifically for this patient population. There are extremely rigid parameters that must be maintained for such patients, along with infection-control protocols. Multiple types of equipment and monitoring systems are placed in this unit.

- The *burn unit* is for patients with multiple types of burns. Patients suffering from thermal, scalding, chemical, or electrical burns need specific treatment.

- The *trauma ICU* is for patients with various types of injuries and diagnoses. The equipment in this unit can range from a simple arterial line to CVVHD to orthopedic traction. Nurses in the trauma ICU must be prepared for any and all types of wounds and patient care.

THE AACN

The AACN is the world's largest specialty nursing organization. It is strongly encouraged that you join a specialty organization. Through an AACN membership, you will have access to continuing education and to journals with evidence-based practice and clinical articles, and the ability to network with critical care nurses through chapter membership and national conferences. Because critical care nursing is constantly changing and evolving, access to current, cutting-edge information is vital. The mission of the AACN is:

Patients and their families rely on nurses at the most vulnerable times of their lives. Acute and critical care nurses rely on AACN for expert knowledge and the influence to fulfill their promise to patients and their families. AACN drives excellence because nothing less is acceptable. (AACN, 2019b)

The AACN has developed several standards that describe the practice and performance of nursing. These standards include:

- AACN Standards for Establishing and Sustaining Healthy Work Environments
- AACN Scope and Standards for Acute and Critical Care Nursing Practice
- AACN Scope and Standards for Acute Care Nurse Practitioner Practice
- AACN Scope and Standards for Acute Care Clinical Nurse Specialist Practice
- AACN TeleICU Nursing Consensus Statement

A healthy work environment is a priority to provide excellent patient care. Healthy work environments foster a culture of trust, collaboration, communication, and teamwork. The AACN's standards for establishing and sustaining a healthy work environment identify six components that are a hallmark of nursing excellence (AACN, 2019a):

1. Skilled communication
2. True collaboration
3. Effective decision-making
4. Appropriate staffing
5. Meaningful recognition
6. Authentic leadership

In addition to outlining standards of care and identifying the essential components of a healthy critical care environment, the AACN also offers certification in critical care nursing. Specialty certification indicates your commitment to continued education and increased knowledge in the care of critically/acutely ill patients. More information on the specialty certification is provided in Chapter 3, Specialty Certification for Critical Care Nurses.

Resources

American Association of Critical-Care Nurses. (2019). *AACN standards.* Retrieved from https://www.aacn.org/nursing-excellence/aacn-standards
American Association of Critical-Care Nurses. (2019). *AACN standards for establishing and sustaining healthy work environments.* Retrieved from https://www.aacn.org/~/media/aacn-website/nursing-excellence/healthy -work-environment/execsum.pdf?la=en

References

American Association of Critical-Care Nurses. (2010, April). *Media resources*. Retrieved from https://www.aacn.org/~/media/aacn-website/newsroom/newsroompresskit.doc?la=en

American Association of Critical-Care Nurses. (2019a). *Healthy work environments*. Retrieved from https://www.aacn.org/nursing-excellence/healthy-work-environments?tab=Patient%20Care

American Association of Critical-Care Nurses. (2019b). *Mission statement*. Retrieved from https://www.aacn.org/about-aacn

2

The Electronic Medical Record and Documentation

Accurate documentation of patient care is essential regardless of the patient care setting. The electronic medical record (EMR) replaces the paper documentation process and is now customary in a majority of healthcare settings. In February 2009, the American Recovery and Reinvestment Act (ARRA) was enacted. The goal of this Act was to modernize the infrastructure within the United States; as part of that goal, the Health Information Technology for Economic and Clinical Health Act (HITECH) required the implementation of the EMR in hospitals and physician offices.

Regardless of the documentation process, clear, concise documentation of patient care and the patient's response is vital.

In this chapter, you will learn:

1. The five steps in the nursing process
2. The basic rules for documenting patient care
3. The definition of malpractice and documentation strategies that can help prevent its occurrence

NURSING STANDARDS OF PRACTICE

Nursing is based on standards that define, guide, and evaluate nursing practice along with its suggested outcomes. The American Nurses Association (ANA) describes six core standards of practice:

1. *Assessment:* Collection of data
2. *Diagnosis:* Analysis of data to determine the nursing diagnosis
3. *Outcome identification:* Identification of expected outcomes specific to the patient and/or situation
4. *Planning:* Development of a plan detailing interventions aimed to achieve expected outcomes
5. *Implementation:* Performance of the interventions noted in the plan of care
6. *Evaluation:* Evaluation of the patient's progress toward the achievement of expected outcomes (ANA, 2015)

THE NURSING PROCESS

The ANA describes the nursing process as the "essential core of practice for the registered nurse." The five steps of the nursing process are as follows:

1. *Assessment:* The gathering of psychosocial, physical, spiritual, economic, and lifestyle factors by:
   a. Interviewing the patient and/or family members
   b. Reviewing past medical history and records
   c. Completing a physical examination and reviewing current patient data
2. *Diagnosis:* The issue on which the nursing care plan is based. The nursing diagnosis is the nurse's clinical judgment regarding the patient's response to actual or possible medical problems. It is based on the assessment.
3. *Planning and outcomes:* The nursing care plan details planning and outcomes by:
   a. Assigning priorities, if the patient has multiple nursing diagnoses
   b. Setting short- and long-term goals that are patient oriented and measurable
   c. Including assessment and diagnosis details
   d. Stating appropriate nursing interventions and corresponding medical orders
   e. Utilizing a standardized or computerized care plan or clinical pathway as a guideline, if appropriate
4. *Implementation:* The performance of nursing care according to the care plan by:

a. Properly documenting the care provided to the patient
b. Performing treatment in a way that minimizes complications and life-threatening issues
c. Involving patients, families, caregivers, and other members of the healthcare team as their abilities and patient safety allow
5. *Evaluation:* The process of evaluating the status of the patient and the effectiveness of the treatment. The plan of care may be modified if warranted.

These five steps drive how a nurse determines, completes, and documents patient care, the patient's response to care, education, and healthcare team interaction.

The American Association of Critical-Care Nurses (AACN) Standards of Care and AACN Scope of Practice further define the critical care nurse's role in quality nursing practice: expected professionalism; education; collegiality; ethical situations; collaboration with the patient, family, and healthcare team; clinical inquiries; utilizing appropriate resources; and leadership (Bell, 2015). Additional information is provided on the AACN website (www.aacn.org) and in *AACN Scope and Standards for Acute and Critical Care Nursing Practice.*

DOCUMENTATION

EMRs and electronic medication administration records (EMARs) are designed to make documentation easier, as they have programs and pages for numerous situations that occur in critical care units. However, documenting all the required assessments, care plans, EMARs, physician orders, and multiple other components can be a daunting task. A nurse must remember the nursing process, liability, safety, and patient care when documenting. It is always necessary to "save," or store, the information after inputting it properly.

Each hospital should have a tech team available 24-7 whose responsibility is to help the staff resolve documentation problems involving EMRs and EMARs.

Fast Facts

A critical care nurse must be aware that despite all the technology employed in the ICU, the rule "If it was not documented, it was not done" still holds true. EMRs and EMARs are the center of communication among nursing staff, medical staff, therapists, the lab, the pharmacy, and all other members of the healthcare team. If something is not documented, it cannot be verified and evaluated properly.

If an item, procedure, complication, patient/family situation, or other activity is not on the EMR, find an appropriate place to add the issue in a free-text location.

MALPRACTICE

Critical care nurses must document all aspects of patient care while following each step of the nursing process in their daily practice. Patient and family education must also be documented. Restraints, physical or chemical, require strict documentation following facility-specific guidelines. The best way to ensure proper patient care and outcomes, while avoiding malpractice issues, is to maintain detail-oriented, appropriate documentation and provide proficient care focused on patient safety and within the scope of critical care nursing practice.

Fast Facts

The four elements of a malpractice case:

1. Professional duty to the patient
2. Breach of such duty
3. Injury caused by the breach
4. Resulting damages

To avoid negligence, as well as malpractice issues, nurses must practice according to the Nurse Practice Act (NPA) of the state in which care is provided. Guidelines can generally be found via the state's board of nursing or board of health. It is important that nurses be familiar with state laws regarding nurses' legal rights, responsibilities, and scope of practice as well as violations, disciplinary actions, and penalties. This knowledge allows nurses to provide competent care for patients to the best of their abilities.

In most cases, the EMR ensures all aspects of care are documented. It provides for allergy cross-checking when entering medication orders, identifies potential medication interactions, provides references for evidence-based practice, and allows easy access to previous records. However, there are still pitfalls that must be identified and guarded against. A few potential areas for error are:

1. Failure to date, time, and sign an entry
2. Lack of documentation for omitted medications and treatments

3. Incomplete or missing documentation
4. Adding late entries
5. Entering information into the wrong chart

It is up to each individual nurse to decide and buy a malpractice insurance policy. Investigate and research the numerous companies that offer such policies to determine which company and policy suit the practitioner.

Being aware of the skill, experience, and expertise level enables a nurse to seek appropriate collaboration, education, training, and/ or assistance when necessary. Following the chain of command when problems arise is important. Asking questions while providing optimal care, education, and outcomes for patients and their family members is key to nursing practice.

Resources

Congress.gov. (2009). American Recovery and Reinvestment Act (ARRA) 2009. Retrieved from https://www.congress.gov/bill/111th-congress/house -bill/1/text

U.S. Department of Health and Human Services. (2009). *Health Information Technology for Economic and Clinical Health (HITECH) Act enforcement interim final rule.* Retrieved from https://www.hhs.gov/hipaa/for -professionals/special-topics/hitech-act-enforcement-interim-final-rule/ index.html

Yoder-Wise, P. S. (2019). *Leading and managing in nursing* (7th ed.). St. Louis, MO: Elsevier.

References

American Nurses Association. (2015). *Nursing: Scope and standards of practice* (3rd ed.). Silver Springs, MD: American Nurses Association.

Bell, L. (2015). *AACN scope and standards for acute and critical care nursing practice.* Aliso Viejo, CA: American Association of Critical-Care Nurses.

3

Specialty Certification for Critical Care Nurses

*Attaining specialty certification in critical care nursing desig-
nates your commitment to continuing education, safe patient
care, and a broader depth of knowledge. Critical care certifications are available for adult, pediatric, and neonatal nurses
and are based on specific patient populations, such as stroke,
transplant, and burn patients. Certification is attained through
successful completion of an exam and maintained through continuing education.*

In this chapter, you will learn:

1. The certifications available for critical care nurses
2. The importance of obtaining a critical care certification
3. The requirements to obtain and maintain a certification

SPECIALTY CERTIFICATIONS IN CRITICAL CARE FOR REGISTERED NURSES

Attaining licensure as an RN denotes an individual's legal ability to safely and competently practice nursing in a designated state.
Attaining specialty certification demonstrates to your employer, col-
leagues, and patients your enhanced knowledge in the specialty area
of critical care nursing and your commitment to patient safety and
national standards of care.

The American Association of Critical-Care Nurses (AACN) offers specialty certification exams. More than 80,000 nurses worldwide are certified as critical care registered nurses (CCRN) in either adult, pediatric, or neonatal nursing. Preparing for and passing one of these exams demonstrates your commitment to excellent patient care, lifelong learning, and continuing education. Specialty certifications include the following:

- CCRN is for nurses providing direct care to acutely and critically ill adult, pediatric, and neonatal patients.
- CCRN-K is for nurses who influence the care delivered to acutely and critically ill adult, pediatric, or neonatal patients but do not primarily or exclusively provide direct care.
- CCRN-E is for nurses working in an intensive care unit telemedicine (tele-ICU) monitoring/caring for acutely and critically ill adult patients from a remote location.
- Progressive Critical Care Nurse (PCCN) certification is for progressive care nurses providing direct care to acutely ill adult patients.
- PCCN-K is for nurses who influence the care delivered to acutely ill adult patients but do not primarily or exclusively provide direct care.

In addition to these specialty certifications, the AACN offers subspecialty certifications. These include the following:

- Cardiac Medicine Certification (CMC) is for nurses providing direct care to acutely and critically ill adult cardiac patients.
- Cardiac Surgery Certification (CSC) is for nurses providing direct care to adult patients during the first 48 hours after cardiac surgery.

CCRN eligibility requirements are:

- Current, unencumbered RN license

- Practice providing direct care to acutely/critically ill patients during the past 2 years with 875 hours in the last year
- The name and contact information of a professional associate for clinical hour verification (AACN, 2019)

SPECIALTY CERTIFICATIONS IN NEUROSCIENCE NURSING

The American Association of Neuroscience Nurses (AANN) also addresses the care of critically ill patients. As the leading authority in neuroscience nursing, the AANN is committed to advancing the science and practice of neuroscience nursing. This vision is accomplished through advocacy, education, certification, and setting standards of care. The AANN provides the following certifications:

- Certified Neuroscience Registered Nurse (CNRN) formally recognizes the attainment and demonstration of a unique body of knowledge necessary for the practice of neuroscience nursing.

    CNRN eligibility requirements are:

  - Current, unencumbered RN license
  - Practice providing direct or indirect patient care in neuroscience nursing for 1 year in the last 3 years with 2,080 hours of patient care

- Stroke Certified Registered Nurse (SCRN) formally recognizes the attainment and demonstration of a unique body of knowledge necessary for the practice of stroke nursing.

    SCRN eligibility requirements are:

  - Current, unencumbered RN license
  - Practice providing direct or indirect stroke care through clinical practice, administration, consultation, or as educator or researcher for 1 year in the last 3 years with 2,080 hours of patient care

CLINICAL TRANSPLANT NURSE CERTIFICATION

The American Board of Transplant Certification offers the Certified Clinical Transplant Nurse (CCTN) exam with the following eligibility requirements:

- One year's experience as an RN
- One year's experience providing care to transplant patients

ADDITIONAL CERTIFICATIONS FOR RNs

Additional certifications are available through the American Nurses Credentialing Center (ANCC). Although these are not specific to critical care, available certifications include:

- Medical/Surgical
- Gastrointestinal
- Cardiovascular
- Informatics
- Gerontological
- Case Management
- Nurse Executive and Nurse Executive Advanced

Obtaining certification identifies you as a committed, professional healthcare provider. After successful completion of the exam, the certification is maintained through documentation of continuing education and a fee. Certifications generally have to be renewed every 2 to 5 years, depending on the organization.

Resources

American Association of Critical-Care Nurses. (n.d.-a). *Board certification*. Retrieved from https://www.aacn.org/certification?tab=First-Time%20Certification

American Association of Critical-Care Nurses. (n.d.-b). *CCRN (Adult)*. Retrieved from https://www.aacn.org/certification/get-certified/ccrn-adult

American Association of Critical-Care Nurses. (n.d.-c). *Frequently asked questions about CCRN certification*. Retrieved from https://www.aacn.org/certification/get-certified/ccrn-frequently-asked-questions

American Association of Neuroscience Nurses. (n.d.). *ABNN certification for CNRN and SCRN*. Retrieved from http://aann.org/education/abnn-certification

American Board of Neuroscience Nursing. (n.d.). *Dates and deadlines*. Retrieved from http://abnncertification.org

American Board for Transplant Certification: https://abtc.net

American Nurses Credentialing Center. (n.d.). *Our certifications*. Retrieved from https://www.nursingworld.org/our-certifications/

Reference

American Association of Critical-Care Nurses. (2019). *CCRN exam handbook*. Retrieved from https://www.aacn.org/~/media/aacn-website/certification/get-certified/handbooks/ccrnexamhandbook.pdf

4

Nurse Self-Care and Wellness in the ICU

The critical care environment can be stressful. It is a fast-paced, ever-changing environment filled with incredible highs and heartbreaking lows. The work, while highly satisfying, can be emotionally taxing and physically demanding. Nurses working in the critical care environment may work an entire 12-hour shift on their feet to meet the care demands of patients and their families, often neglecting self-care, such as nutrition and mental health.

To maintain high levels of care, all nurses, including critical care nurses, must practice self-care techniques that become a habit. If not, fatigue and burnout may ensue.

In this chapter, you will learn:

1. Self-care guidelines for nurses working in a critical care environment
2. The American Nurses Association's (ANA) support and resources for healthy living
3. Self-care habits to improve physical and mental health

SELF-CARE FOR CRITICAL CARE NURSES

Working in the field of nursing is difficult and demanding, but it is very rewarding. Critical care nursing has adrenaline highs and corresponding lows often surpassing those of other nursing practice areas. Critical care nurses must learn how to handle and relieve stress to perform their job effectively.

It is crucial that nurses take the time to care for themselves. If not, with mental fatigue and burnout, their physical health may suffer. The ANA declared 2017 the Year of the Healthy Nurse: Balance Your Life for a Healthier You! The yearlong focus on nurses' self-care reflects the physical and mental challenges they face every day. The practices recommended by the ANA should become a part of nurses' daily activities in order to provide optimum care to others. Resources included:

- Worksite wellness and worker well-being
- Nutrition
- Happiness
- Mental health
- Healthy sleep

As a follow-up to this initiative, the ANA launched the Healthy Nurse, Healthy Nation Grand Challenge. Its purpose is to transform the health of the nation by improving the health of nurses. As part of this initiative, over 9,000 nurses and nursing students responded to the HealthyNurse® Survey that focused on the five domains of health: physical activity, quality of life, rest, nutrition, and safety. Important takeaways from this survey are:

- Physical activity: 45% of the respondents indicated they never participated in vigorous/aerobic activity.
- Quality of life: 70% rated their overall health as good or very good.
- Rest: 14% reported falling asleep/dozing off while driving within the previous 30 days.
- Nutrition: Healthy food choices were available to 54%, while 55% reported that healthy food was expensive.
- Safety: Safety metrics included workplace safety, risks, safe patient handling, bullying and workplace violence, and workload (see Box 4.1).

Critical care nurses work as a team, so you need to watch out for each other, both physically and mentally. A recent study by Cordoza et al. (2018) revealed that taking a break outdoors in a garden compared to indoor-only breaks may decrease the risk for burnout. Simply stepping away from the critical care unit and getting some fresh air may recharge and prepare you for the remainder of the shift.

With the majority of critical care nurses working 12-hour shifts, the quality and quantity of sleep may suffer. Fatigue due to lack of sleep may lead to decreased energy and alertness, which may result in a patient care–related error. Further, sleep deprivation is linked to obesity, hypertension, and mood disorder (Francis, 2018). Conversely,

BOX 4.1   SAFETY FOR THE CRITICAL CARE NURSE

Environment/workplace: Over 75% were not worried about their personal safety at work.

Risks: The most common safety risk was stress at work.

Injuries/safe patient handling: 9% reported being injured at work, and 77% of them reported the injury. Over half the respondents had musculoskeletal pain while at work. Almost 75% had access to safe patient handling devices.

Bullying and workplace violence: 64% of the respondents were comfortable reporting bullying at work. Being verbally or physically threatened by a patient or family member was reported by almost 30%.

Workload: 26% reported being assigned a higher workload than they were comfortable taking.

Source: American Nurses Association. (n.d.). *Healthy Nurse, Healthy Nation*. Retrieved from https://www.nursingworld.org/practice-policy/work-environ ment/health-safety/healthy-nurse-healthy-nation/

well-rested nurses are energetic and have better stamina, judgment, and concentration.

Journaling may also relieve stress (Dimitroff, 2018). Through journaling, nurses may find a private outlet to express their thoughts and emotions and meditate on both positive and negative patient care experiences. Research has demonstrated that journaling provides a reflective learning experience that helps reduce blood pressure, decrease absenteeism, and improve mood. Further, it may provide an opportunity to develop critical thinking skills.

Fast Facts

Strategies to Relieve Stress

1. Stay hydrated and eat well-balanced meals.
2. Exercise and maintain flexibility.
3. Get 7–8 hours of sleep daily.
4. Separate work and home life; spend off-duty time with family and friends.
5. Maintain a positive outlook.

(continued)

(continued)

6. Participate in hobbies outside of work.
7. Maintain a sense of humor.
8. Take 3 seconds to just breathe.
9. Discuss concerns about patients, coworkers, and/or doctors with the nurse manager.
10. Seek counseling, if needed, to handle grief, emotions, and stress.

In addition to following a healthy diet and managing stress while remaining physically and emotionally fit, ICU nurses should see their own physicians at least once a year, stay up-to-date on immunizations, and receive annual flu shots.

By actively providing self-care, nurses improve the quality of care they provide to their patients and loved ones. All the strategies mentioned will help keep stress at a minimum; however, there is one key to performing well and making the best decisions while on the job: Do what is best for the patient. By honoring this mantra, nurses will ask questions when needed, seek appropriate consultation, and provide the right type of care, all while exhibiting great nursing skills and protecting their licenses.

References

American Nurses Association. (n.d.). *Healthy Nurse, Healthy Nation*. Retrieved from https://www.nursingworld.org/practice-policy/work-environment/health-safety/healthy-nurse-healthy-nation/

Cordoza, M., Ulrich, R. S., Manulik, B. J., Gardiner, S. K., Fitzpatrick, P. S., Hazen, T. M., . . . Perkins, R. S. (2018). Impact of nurses taking daily work breaks in a hospital garden on burnout. *American Journal of Critical Care, 27*(6), 508–512. doi:10.4037/ajcc2018131

Dimitroff, L. J. (2018). Journaling: A valuable tool for registered nurses. *American Nurse Today, 13*(11), 27.

Francis, R. (2018). Nurse fatigue: A shared responsibility. *American Nurse Today, 13*(11), 26.

II

Critical Care by Body System

5

Neurological Critical Care

Patients in the neurological critical care unit (neuro-ICU) may be admitted for a variety of reasons, including planned and unplanned cranial surgery; trauma, including head and/or spinal injury; strokes; seizures; or other medical conditions. Having a thorough knowledge of neurological assessment and monitoring techniques is essential regardless of the primary admitting diagnosis.

In this chapter, you will learn:

1. How to conduct a neurological assessment
2. Specific neurological assessments in the neuro-ICU
3. How to care for patients with specific neurological conditions
4. Intracranial pressure (ICP) monitoring

NEUROLOGICAL ASSESSMENT

The completion of a comprehensive neurological assessment is an important aspect of caring for a patient in the neuroICU. There are five major components of the neurological assessment:

1. Level of consciousness (LOC)
2. Motor function
3. Pupillary function
4. Respiratory function
5. Vital signs

Table 5.1

Levels of Consciousness	
Term	**Responsiveness**
Alert	Normal. Responds with minimal stimuli.
Awake	Somewhat confused on awakening, but fully oriented.
Confused	Oriented to person, but not time/place. Decreased attention span.
Delirious	Disoriented to time, place, and person. May have visual and auditory hallucinations.
Lethargic	Drowsy but follows simple commands. Requires increased stimulation to respond.
Obtunded	Indifferent to external stimulation. Responds with a word or two.
Stuporous	Responds to vigorous and continuous external stimuli. Limited spontaneous movement.
Comatose	Reflexive posturing or no response to any stimulus.

Source: Adapted from Morton, P. G., & Fontaine, D. K. (2018). *Critical care nursing: A holistic approach* (11th ed.). Philadelphia, PA: Wolters Kluwer; and Urden, L. D., Stacy, K. M., & Lough, M. E. (2020). *Priorities in critical care nursing* (8th ed.). St. Louis, MO: Elsevier

One of the first key assessments is to determine the patient's LOC. It may be classified as described in Table 5.1.

The Glasgow Coma Scale (GCS) is a scoring system used to evaluate the LOC (Exhibit 5.1). A score of less than 7 indicates a coma.

All members of the healthcare team use these initial assessments to determine the patient's baseline neurological status. Numerous

Exhibit 5.1

The Glasgow Coma Scale	
Response	**Score**
Eye Opening:	
• Spontaneous: blinks/opens eyes without stimulation	4
• To verbal stimulus or command	3
• To pain only	2
• No response to stimulus	1
Verbal Response:	
• Oriented	5
• Confused, but answers questions	4
• Inappropriate words	3

(continued)

Exhibit 5.1

The Glasgow Coma Scale (*continued*)

Response	Score
• Incomprehensible sounds	2
• None (a *T* may be noted to acknowledge trach/ETT)	1
Motor Response:	
• Obeys/follows commands	6
• Localizes: tries to remove stimulus	5
• Withdraws from stimulus	4
• Abnormal flexion, decorticate posturing	3
• Abnormal extension, decerebrate posturing	2
• No movement in response to stimulus	1
Note: A score of 15 is considered normal.	

ETT, endotracheal tube.

Source: Adapted from Burns, S. M., & Delgado, S. A. (2019). *AACN essentials of critical care nursing* (4th ed.). New York, NY: McGraw-Hill; Diepenbrock, N. H. (2016). *Quick reference to critical care* (5th ed.). Philadelphia, PA: Wolters Kluwer; Morton, P. G., & Fontaine, D. K. (2018). *Critical care nursing: A holistic approach* (11th ed.). Philadelphia, PA: Wolters Kluwer; and Urden, L. D., Stacy, K. M., & Lough, M. E. (2020). *Priorities in critical care nursing* (8th ed.). St. Louis, MO: Elsevier.

tests can uncover the cause of changes in neurological function and assist with determining the course of treatment.

In addition to routine lab tests of arterial blood gas (ABG) analysis, comprehensive metabolic panel, drug screens, urinalysis, and basic x-rays, imaging studies may be ordered, as shown in Table 5.2.

Table 5.2

Diagnostic and Imaging Tests for Determining Neurological Status

Diagnostic/Imaging Test	Potential Diagnosis
CT scan with and without contrast	Hemorrhage Aneurysm or vascular abnormality Stroke (infarction) Infection Tumors
PET scan SPECT Nuclear medicine study conducted during CT scan	Determine the functionality of blood flow movement within the brain Distribution of metabolites into tumors

(*continued*)

Table 5.2

Diagnostic and Imaging Tests for Determining Neurological Status (continued)	
Diagnostic/Imaging Test	**Potential Diagnosis**
MRI MRA	Cerebral aneurysm, embolic, and infarct Hydrocephalus Infection Trauma: skull fracture Tumor Vertebral artery dissection
Transcranial Doppler	Determine intracranial blood flow Subarachnoid hemorrhage Stroke
Myelography/myelogram	Evaluate spinal cord, nerve roots, and meninges Utilized if the patient is unable to undergo an MRI/MRA

SPECT, single-photon emission tomography; MRA, magnetic resonance angiography.

Additional diagnostic tests include lumbar puncture with cerebrospinal fluid (CSF) analysis and nerve conduction studies.

DIAGNOSES

Cerebrovascular Accident (Stroke)

A cerebrovascular accident (CVA), or stroke, is an interruption of the blood flow to the brain. Sometimes referred to as a "brain attack," CVAs

Exhibit 5.2

National Institutes of Health Stroke Scale		
Category	**Title**	**Response and Score**
1A	Level of consciousness	0—Alert 1—Drowsy 2—Obtunded 3—Coma/unresponsive
1B	Orientation questions (2)	0—Answers both questions correctly 1—Answers one question correctly 2—Answers neither question correctly
1C	Response to commands (2)	0—Obeys both commands correctly 1—Obeys one command correctly 2—Performs neither command

(continued)

Exhibit 5.2

National Institutes of Health Stroke Scale Assessment (*continued*)

Category	Title	Response and Score
2	Gaze	0—Normal horizontal movements 1—Partial gaze palsy 2—Complete gaze palsy
3	Visual fields	0—No visual field defect 1—Partial hemianopia 2—Complete hemianopia 3—Bilateral hemianopia
4	Facial movement	0—Normal 1—Minor facial weakness 2—Partial facial weakness 3—Complete unilateral palsy
5	Motor function (arm) a. Right b. Left	0—No drift 1—Drift before 5 sec 2—Falls before 10 sec 3—No effort against gravity 4—No movement
6	Motor function (leg) a. Right b. Left	0—No drift 1—Drift before 5 sec 2—Falls before 5 sec 3—No effort against gravity 4—No movement
7	Limb ataxia	0—No ataxia 1—Ataxia in one limb 2—Ataxia in two limbs
8	Sensory	0—No sensory loss 1—Mild sensory loss 2—Severe sensory loss
9	Language	0—Normal 1—Mild aphasia 2—Severe aphasia 3—Mute or global aphasia
10	Articulation	0—Normal 1—Mild dysarthria 2—Severe dysarthria
11	Extinction or inattention	0—Absent 1—Mild 2—Severe

Source: Adapted from Diepenbrock, N. H. (2016). *Quick reference to critical care* (5th ed.). Philadelphia, PA: Wolters Kluwer, and Kothari, R. U., Pancioli, A., Liu, T., & Beroderick, J. (1999). Cincinnati Prehospital Stroke Scale: Reproducibility and validity. *Annals of Emergency Medicine, 33*(4), 373–378. doi:10.1016/s0196-0644(99)70299-4

may be *ischemic* or *hemorrhagic*. Strokes are the fifth leading cause of death in the United States. Those surviving a stroke may face varying levels of disability. The National Institutes of Health Stroke Scale (NIHSS) is an assessment tool that quantifies stroke-related neurological deficits (Exhibit 5.2). The scale is used to evaluate the acuity and severity of a stroke, help determine treatment, and predict outcomes.

Ischemic Stroke

Causes: Seventy-five to 85% of all strokes are ischemic and are caused by a thrombotic or an embolic event. The accumulation of atherosclerotic plaques may lead to a thrombus that obstructs the flow of blood to the brain. The most common sites for atherosclerotic plaques are the common carotid arteries, middle and anterior cerebral arteries, and vertebral arteries.

Embolic strokes are the result of a small embolus that forms in either the heart or the lower circulation and travels to the brain, lodging in a small artery and obstructing the blood flow to the brain. Emboli may be from blood clots, air, fat, or tumor fragments. The most common form is the result of chronic atrial fibrillation, valvular disease, and cardiomyopathy.

Signs and Symptoms: A sudden onset of focal neurological changes lasting greater than 24 hours occurs. Common neurological symptoms include:

- Hemiparesis: weakness/paralysis on one side of the body
- Aphasia: inability to speak or slurred speech
- Hemianopia: visual changes

Depending on the location and extent of ischemia in the brain, the following symptoms may be noted:

- Change in LOC
- Seizure
- Hypoxia
- Elevated ICP

Interventions: After confirmation of the type of stroke, fibrinolytic therapy with recombinant tissue plasminogen activator (rtPA) is recommended. This medication must be administered within 3 to 4.5 hours of the onset of symptoms. The medication will dissolve the clot, allowing for reperfusion of the brain tissue. Patients must be carefully assessed according to hospital-specific protocols prior to administration of the medication.

Hemorrhagic Stroke

Causes: Occurring less frequently than ischemic strokes, hemorrhagic strokes are the result of hypertensive vascular disease, a ruptured aneurysm, or an arteriovenous malformation. The bleeding may be classified as intracerebral or subarachnoid (SAH), with intracerebral occurring approximately 67% of the time. Care of the patient with a hemorrhagic stroke is different from that an ischemic stroke.

Signs and Symptoms: Patients with a hemorrhagic stroke often complain of a sudden and severe headache. The patient may complain of the "worst headache of my life." Other symptoms include nausea and vomiting, change in LOC, and seizures. Specific neurological signs will vary based on the location and extent of the hemorrhage.

Interventions: Confirm the type of stroke with a CT scan. Hemorrhagic strokes may be devastating and have a 30-day mortality rate of 44% to 75% depending on location and extent (Morton & Fontaine, 2018). Based on the presentation, the patient may require intubation and mechanical ventilation. Other therapies will be directed at maintaining and/or lowering the ICP with blood pressure control, osmotic diuretics, hyperventilation via the ventilator, and ventricular drainage. Continuous ICP monitoring may be implemented.

Fast Facts

- Utilize the NIHSS scale to evaluate and monitor patients with stroke.
- The Cincinnati Prehospital Stroke Scale (CPSS) is a quick and simple assessment tool (Exhibit 5.3).
- Patients receiving rtPA should not receive any other form of anticoagulants for at least 24 hours.
  - This includes aspirin, heparin, and warfarin.
- CT scan must be completed prior to administering rtPA.

Transient Ischemic Attack

A transient ischemic attack (TIA) is the development of stroke symptoms that resolve within minutes and without lasting neurological effects. TIAs may be a warning or precursor to a stroke and require extensive assessment and evaluation. Sometimes referred to as a

Exhibit 5.3

The Cincinnati Prehospital Stroke Scale		
	Normal	**Abnormal**
Facial droop smile	Equal	One side does not move; uneven
Arm drift	Both arms move equally	One arm drifts
Speech	Clear and correct	Slurred or inappropriate

If one of the three parameters is abnormal, there is a 72% chance the individual is having a stroke.

Source: Adapted from Diepenbrock, N. H. (2016). *Quick reference to critical care* (5th ed.). Philadelphia, PA: Wolters Kluwer; Kothari, R. U., Pancioli, A., Liu, T., & Beroderick, J. (1999). Cincinnati Prehospital Stroke Scale: Reproducibility and validity. *Annals of Emergency Medicine, 33*(4), 373–378. doi:10.1016/s0196-0644(99)70299-4; National Institute of Health (nih.gov); and Urden, L. D., Stacy, K. M., & Lough, M. E. (2020). *Priorities in critical care nursing* (8th ed.). St. Louis, MO: Elsevier

"ministroke," approximately 15% of strokes are preceded by a TIA (American Stroke Association, n.d.).

Causes

A small blood clot blocks the artery for a short period of time. The clot may be dissolved by the body's natural anticoagulant action or pushed out of the way.

Signs and Symptoms

Signs and symptoms are similar to ischemic stroke symptoms but only last for a short period of time and are then resolved.

Interventions

Although the patient may currently not present with signs and symptoms of a stroke, a full assessment and diagnostic tests must be performed.

Intracranial Aneurysm

A weakening of the arterial wall that results in a ballooning effect or distention is an aneurysm. Aneurysms may be the result of long-standing hypertension resulting in degenerative arterial lesions or congenital. Intracranial aneurysms typically occur within the circle of Willis. A rupture of the aneurysm results in SAH.

Causes

The exact cause of aneurysms is not well understood, but current evidence suggests a combination of acquired and genetic traits. Acquired conditions include hypertension, cigarette smoking, traumatic brain injury, and sepsis. Other conditions that are associated with intracranial aneurysm include Marfan's syndrome, coarctation of the aorta, polycystic kidney disease, and system lupus erythematosus (Morton & Fontaine, 2018).

Signs and Symptoms

Individuals with aneurysms do not display signs and symptoms until the aneurysm leaks or bursts. A leaking aneurysm may cause warning signs, including headache, lethargy, neck pain, a "noise in the head," and dysfunction of the optic, oculomotor, and trigeminal cranial nerves. A rupture of the aneurysm is described as "the worst headache of my life," with ensuing deterioration of neurological status. Severity of symptoms depends on the location and extent of bleeding.

Interventions

Minimal stimulation of the patient is crucial to prevent rebleeding, along with maintaining a quiet environment, providing stool softeners to prevent straining, and limiting visitors.
Additional measures include:

- Mild analgesics for headache. Opioids are avoided because they may mask neurological changes.
- Antipyretics, usually acetaminophen, for fever that is the result of blood in the subarachnoid space.

Surgical intervention is required if the aneurysm is in an accessible location. If possible, a clip is placed around the neck of the aneurysm.

Seizures/Status Epilepticus

A seizure is an uncontrolled electrical discharge of neurons in the brain that results from an imbalance of excitatory and inhibitory impulses. Status epilepticus refers to a continued seizure activity lasting greater than 5 minutes.

Causes

Seizures may be caused by a variety of conditions, including:

- Trauma
- Hemorrhage

- Central nervous system (CNS) infection
- Tumor
- Systemic causes:
  - Hypoxia
  - Hypoglycemia
  - Drug overdose
  - Drug or alcohol withdrawal

Signs and Symptoms

The signs and symptoms exhibited by the patient are dependent on the cause of the seizure and may vary from a loss of consciousness to fully sustained tonic-clonic muscle jerking. Focal seizures, once termed simple partial, are limited to one area or hemisphere of the brain. Generalized seizures, previously referred to as grand mal and/or petit mal, affect both hemispheres of the brain. Further, generalized seizures may be classified as follows:

- Absence: Sudden lapse of consciousness lasting 3 to 30 seconds
- Myoclonic: Sudden brief muscle jerking
- Atonic: Sudden loss of muscle tone
- Clonic: Rhythmic muscle jerking
- Tonic: Sustained muscle contraction
- Tonic-clonic: Varies between sustained contractions and muscle jerking

Interventions

Maintaining patient's safety and preventing injury is one of the first interventions. Airway management is crucial, and this is accomplished through controlling or managing the seizure. Positioning the patient in a side-lying posture will help prevent aspiration. Do not place anything in the patient's mouth and provide supplemental oxygen. After the seizure is controlled and the patient is safe, the process of determining the underlying cause begins. Refer to Box 5.1 for first-line medications.

CRANIOTOMY

Craniotomy is the surgical procedure to access portions of the brain/CNS. Typically, craniotomies are performed to remove tumors, hematomas, decompress the cerebral space, or clip or remove an aneurysm. Depending on the initial diagnosis and extent of the surgery, the patient will require critical care monitoring, including:

- GCS
- LOC
- ICP
- Cerebral perfusion pressure (CPP)
- Ventriculostomy for CSF drainage

BOX 5.1 MEDICATIONS FOR SEIZURE MANAGEMENT

Fast-acting anticonvulsants:

Lorazepam (Ativan): 0.1 mg/kg up to 4 mg per dose IV; no faster than 2 mg/min; repeat in 5–10 minutes

Midazolam (Versed): 0.2 mg/kg IM to a maximum dose of 10 mg

Diazepam (Valium): 0.15 mg/kg IV up to 10 mg per dose; no faster than 5 mg/min; may repeat in 5 minutes

Long-acting anticonvulsants:

Phenytoin (Dilantin): Loading: 20 mg/kg IV; no faster than 50 mg/min; may give additional 5–10 mg/kg 10 minutes after loading dose

Phenobarbital: Loading: 20 mg/kg IV; no faster than 50–100 mg/min; may give additional 5–10 mg/kg 10 minutes after loading dose

Fosphenytoin (Cerebyx): 20 mg/kg IV; no faster than 150 mg/min; may give additional 5 mg/kg 10 minutes after loading dose

Source: Adapted from Burns, S. M., & Delgado, S. A. (2019). *AACN essentials of critical care nursing* (4th ed.). New York, NY: McGraw-Hill; Jones, J., & Fix, B. (2015). *Critical care notes: Clinical pocket guide* (2nd ed.). Philadelphia, PA: F.A. Davis; Morton, P. G., & Fontaine, D. K. (2018). *Critical care nursing: A holistic approach* (11th ed.). Philadelphia, PA: Wolters Kluwer

Fast Facts

An ICP reading from a ventricular catheter is fairly easy:

1. Zero and relevel the transducer with the external auditory canal, or as ordered.
2. Close the CSF drainage system, if applicable.
3. Perform an ICP reading at end-expiration.

(continued)

(continued)

Source: Adapted from Ehlers, J. (Ed.). (2007). *AACN's quick reference guide to critical care nursing procedures.* St. Louis, MO: Saunders Elsevier.

Resources

Bladh, V. L. (2019). *Davis's comprehensive manual of laboratory and diagnostic tests with nursing interventions* (8th ed.). Philadelphia, PA: F.A. Davis.

Boling, B., & Keinath, K. (2018). Acute ischemic stroke. *AACN Advanced Critical Care, 29*(2), 152–162. doi:10.4037/aacnacc2018483. Retrieved from http://acc.aacnjournals.org/content/29/2/152

Hinkle, J. L., & Cheever, K. H. (2017). *Brunner & Suddarth's handbook of laboratory and diagnostic tests* (3rd ed.). Philadelphia, PA: Wolters Kluwer.

NIH Stroke Scale International. (n.d.). *The International Network.* Retrieved from http://www.nihstrokescale.org

References

American Stroke Association. (n.d.). *TIA (transient ischemic attack).* Retrieved from https://www.strokeassociation.org/STROKEORG/About Stroke/TypesofStroke/TIA/Transient-Ischemic-Attack-TIA_UCM_492003 _SubHomePage.jsp

Burns, S. M., & Delgado, S. A. (2019). *AACN essentials of critical care nursing* (4th ed.). New York, NY: McGraw-Hill.

Diepenbrock, N. H. (2016). *Quick reference to critical care* (5th ed.). Philadelphia, PA: Wolters Kluwer.

Ehlers, J. (Ed.). (2007). *AACN's quick reference guide to critical care nursing procedures.* St. Louis, MO: Saunders Elsevier.

Jones, J., & Fix, B. (2015). *Critical care notes: Clinical pocket guide* (2nd ed.). Philadelphia, PA: F.A. Davis.

Kirchman, M. (2010). *Intracranial pressure monitoring and drainage of cerebrospinal fluid via ventricular catheter.* Retrieved from www.home.smh .com/sections/servicesprocedures/medlib/nursing/NursPandP/crc10 _intracranial_041910.pdf

Kothari, R. U., Pancioli, A., Liu, T., & Beroderick, J. (1999). Cincinnati Prehospital Stroke Scale: Reproducibility and validity. *Annals of Emergency Medicine, 33*(4), 373–378. doi:10.1016/s0196-0644 (99)70299-4

Morton, P. G., & Fontaine, D. K. (2018). *Critical care nursing: A holistic approach* (11th ed.). Philadelphia, PA: Wolters Kluwer.

Nettina, S. M. (2010). *Lippincott manual of nursing practice* (9th ed.). Ambler, PA: Wolters Kluwer Health, Lippincott Williams & Wilkins.

Stillwell, S. B. (2006). *Mosby's critical care nursing reference* (4th ed.). St. Louis, MO: Mosby Elsevier.

Urden, L. D., Stacy, K. M., & Lough, M. E. (2020). *Priorities in critical care nursing* (8th ed.). St. Louis, MO: Elsevier.

Wyckoff, M., Houghton, D., & LePage, C. (Eds.). (2009). *Critical care concepts, role, and practice for the acute care nurse practitioner.* New York, NY: Springer Publishing Company.

6

Respiratory Critical Care

Regardless of the critical care environment, management of the airway and the respiratory system is a priority. The vast majority of patients in a critical care setting receive supplemental oxygen through either a simple nasal cannula or a more complex ventilator. Assessment and airway management are vital.

In this chapter, you will learn:

1. How to conduct a respiratory assessment
2. How to care for patients with specific respiratory conditions
3. Arterial blood gas (ABG) interpretation
4. Various methods of providing supplemental oxygen and supporting the airway
5. Various ventilator modes and settings

RESPIRATORY ASSESSMENT

Completion of a comprehensive respiratory assessment is an important aspect of caring for a patient in any critical/acute care setting. The major components of the respiratory assessment are:

1. Tongue and sublingual areas
2. Respiratory rate and effort
3. Chest wall configuration
4. Breath sounds
5. ABG interpretation

Observe the tongue and sublingual areas for cyanosis that may indicate hypoxemia. Carefully observe the patient's respiratory rate and effort while at rest, being sure to monitor the rhythm, symmetry, and quality of effort. Then observe the chest wall configuration with a focus on the anteroposterior (AP) diameter and any structural deviations. Auscultation of breath sounds will reveal any abnormalities that indicate the presence of a pathological process in the lungs. Finally, ABGs will provide an indication of the patient's ability to oxygenate and remove carbon dioxide.

DIAGNOSES

Pneumonia

Community acquired pneumonia (CAP) is an inflammatory process of the lung parenchyma caused by an infectious agent. Hospitalized patients on mechanical ventilation may develop ventilator acquired pneumonia (VAP). VAP is preventable and is an indication of the quality of care provided in the critical care unit.

Causes

Severe CAP occurs outside the hospital setting. It will require admission to the ICU. Common pathogens include:

- *Streptococcus pneumoniae*
- *Legionella* species
- *Haemophilus influenzae*
- *Staphylococcus aureus*

Signs and Symptoms

Initially, the patient may present with dyspnea, fever, and a cough that may or may not be productive. Auscultation of the lung fields will reveal coarse crackles. Progressive CAP will result in confusion, disorientation, tachypnea, hypoxemia, uremia, leukopenia, hypothermia, and hypotension.

See Exhibit 6.1 for the CURB-65 Tool to determine initial treatment.

Interventions

Patient care includes antibiotic therapy, oxygen therapy if hypoxemia is present, mechanical ventilation, fluid management, and nutritional support. Oxygen therapy will be guided by patient status and ABG results. Bronchodilators and mucolytics may also be prescribed.

Exhibit 6.1

CURB-65 Tool for Initial Treatment of Community Acquired Pneumonia (CAP)

CURB-65 Tool for Determining the Initial Treatment of Adults Aged ≥65 With CAP (one point for each positive finding)

- Confusion, disorientation
- Urea: >7 mm/L
- Respiratory rate: >30 breaths/min
- Blood pressure: SBP <9 mmHg or DBP <60 mmHg
- Age: ≥65

Score:

0–1 = Outpatient treatment
2–3 = Inpatient treatment (consider ICU admission if score is 3)
4–5 = ICU admission

DBP, diastolic blood pressure; SBP, systolic blood pressure.

Source: Morton, P.G., & Fontaine, D.K. (2018). *Critical care nursing: A holistic approach* (11th ed.). Philadelphia, PA: Wolters Kluwer.

Fast Facts

VAP Prevention Strategies

VAP rates are indicative of the quality of care provided to patients on mechanical ventilation. It is estimated that a single VAP will increase costs by $20,000 to $40,000 and increase the length of stay by 4 to 12 days. Strategies to prevent VAP include the following:

- Maintain hand hygiene.
- Keep the head of the bed at 30° to 45° unless contraindicated.
- Provide oral care every 2 hours, with a chlorhexidine gluconate rinse with suctioning every 12 hours. Brush teeth, gums, and tongue every 12 hours.
- Provide moisture to oral mucosa and lips every 2 to 4 hours.
- Utilize an endotracheal tube with the capability to provide continuous low suctioning of the glottic area (above the cuff).
- Use a closed ventilation system.
- Use sterile technique for suctioning.
- Provide nutritional support.

(continued)

(continued)

- Remove invasive devices as soon as possible. Assess weaning readiness every day.

Source: Adapted from American Association of Critical-Care Nurses. (2017). Oral care for acutely and critically ill patients. *Critical Care Nurse, 37*(3), e19–e21. doi:10 .4037/ccn2017179. Retrieved from https://www.aacn.org/~/media/aacn-website/ clincial-resources/practice-alerts/oralcarepractalert2017.pdf

Acute Lung Failure

Also referred to as acute respiratory failure, acute lung failure (ALF) is characterized by the inability of the respiratory system to maintain adequate gas exchange. Over half the patients in the critical care unit develop ALF, and there is a 30% to 40% mortality rate.

Causes

ALF is usually a response to another physiological condition that causes a change in the performance of the respiratory system. The causes include injury to the chest wall, lungs, or airways; pulmonary disease; or a complication after surgery. These complications include atelectasis, pulmonary edema, pulmonary embolism, and pneumonia.

Signs and Symptoms

Patients developing ALF will demonstrate hypoxemia or hypercapnia (see Table 6.1).

In addition to the changes in ABGs, patients will also have tachypnea, dyspnea, tachycardia, restlessness, confusion, diaphoresis, and abnormal breath sounds. As the condition deteriorates, the patient will demonstrate somnolence, cyanosis, and loss of consciousness.

Table 6.1

Signs of Hypoxemia or Hypercapnia in Patients Developing Acute Lung Failure	
Hypoxemia	**Hypercapnia**
PaO_2 <50 mmHg	$PaCO_2$ >50 mmHg and pH <7.25

Interventions

Immediate intervention is required to improve and promote adequate gas exchange:

- Provide supplemental oxygen via a high flow nasal cannula or face mask.
- Administer bronchodilators and suction, and place the patient in a high Fowler's position.
- Correct the underlying cause of respiratory failure.
- Prepare for immediate intubation and mechanical ventilation if the patient is not responding to supplemental oxygenation.

Acute Respiratory Distress Syndrome

Noncardiac pulmonary edema is caused by increased alveolar-capillary membrane permeability. Generally, acute respiratory distress syndrome (ARDS) is a complication of multiple organ dysfunction syndrome. The increased permeability of the alveolar-capillary bed will lead to interstitial and alveolar leak, resulting in decreased lung compliance. Decreased lung compliance causes hypoventilation and hypercapnia with severe hypoxemia.

Causes

ARDS may be caused by primary or secondary factors. See Table 6.2.

Table 6.2

Primary and Secondary Factors for ARDS

Primary Factors	Secondary Factors
Near drowning	Sepsis
Inhalation of smoke or toxic substance	Fat emboli
Pneumonia	Pancreatitis
Aspiration	Trauma
Pulmonary contusion	Hypovolemic shock associated with trauma or sepsis
	DIC
	Massive blood transfusion

DIC, disseminated intravascular coagulation.

Source: Adapted from Burns, S. M., & Delgado, S. A. (2019). *AACN essentials of critical care nursing* (4th ed.). New York, NY: McGraw-Hill; Morton, P. G., & Fontaine, D. K. (2018). *Critical care nursing: A holistic approach* (11th ed.). Philadelphia, PA: Wolters Kluwer; Urden, L. D., Stacy, K. M., & Lough, M. E. (2020). *Priorities in critical care nursing* (8th ed.). St. Louis, MO: Elsevier.

Signs and Symptoms

The development of signs and symptoms will progress based on the initial insult and causative factors. Initially, patients will develop dyspnea, tachypnea, tachycardia, anxiety, and chest pain. The ABGs will continue to worsen, requiring an increased fraction of inspired oxygen (FiO_2). The chest x-ray will reveal diffuse bilateral pulmonary infiltrates, sometimes referred to as a "whiteout."

Interventions

Intubation and mechanical ventilation are required to support the patient while treating the underlying cause. Advanced methods of mechanical ventilation are required to promote adequate gas exchange. Extracorporeal membrane oxygenation (ECMO) may be utilized in select patients.

Acute Pulmonary Embolism

Acute pulmonary embolism is a thrombus or thrombi obstructing the pulmonary artery or the pulmonary vasculature.

Causes

Acute pulmonary embolism is usually the result of deep vein thrombosis (DVT) in the legs. Other types of emboli include air, fat from a long-bone fracture, amniotic fluid, tumors, septic thrombi, and vegetation on the heart valves.

Signs and Symptoms

Symptoms will vary depending on the size of the thrombus and the location in the pulmonary vasculature. Patients may present with increasing dyspnea or hemodynamic collapse. Additional signs and symptoms include tachypnea, chest pain, wheezing, crackles, cyanosis, cardiac dysrhythmias, tachycardia, and hypotension.

Interventions

Provide supplemental oxygen by mask or intubation, and ventilation depending on the patient's hemodynamic status. Initiate heparin with a bolus followed by infusion per hospital protocol. Initiate thrombolytic medications as directed. Provide hemodynamic support as indicated. Prepare for embolectomy.

Respiratory Acidosis and Alkalosis

Respiratory acidosis (excess CO_2 retention) causes include hypoventilation due to pulmonary, cardiac, drug overdose, injury, obesity, abdominal distention, and postoperative pain.

Table 6.3

ABG Interpretation for Respiratory Acidosis and Alkalosis			
	pH 7.35–7.45	pCO₂ 35–45	HCO₃ 22–25
Respiratory acidosis	<7.35	>45	WNL
Respiratory alkalosis	>7.45	<35	WNL

WNL, within normal limits.

Fast Facts

ABG Interpretation

Normal

pH	7.35	
pCO₂	35 to 45 mmHg	
pO₂	85 to 95 mmHg	
HCO₃	22 to 25 mEq/L	

Respiratory alkalosis causes include hyperventilation due to anxiety, pain, respiratory stimulation from drugs, fever, hypoxia, and gram-negative bacteremia.

ABG interpretation for respiratory acidosis and alkalosis is described in Table 6.3.

Metabolic Acidosis and Alkalosis

Metabolic acidosis (HCO₃ loss, acid retention) causes include bicarbonate loss due to diarrhea, kidney disease, hepatic disease, diabetes, hypoxia, shock, and drug intoxication.

Table 6.4

ABG Interpretation for Metabolic Acidosis and Alkalosis			
	pH 7.35–7.45	pCO₂ 35–45	HCO₃ 22–25
Metabolic acidosis	<7.35	WNL	<22
Metabolic alkalosis	>7.45	WNL	>22

Metabolic alkalosis (HCO_3 retention, acid loss) causes include loss of hydrochloric acid from prolonged vomiting or gastric suctioning, excess renal secretion of potassium, and excessive alkali ingestion.

ABG interpretation for respiratory acidosis and alkalosis is described in Table 6.4.

SUPPLEMENTAL OXYGENATION METHODS

Depending on the patient's status, supplemental oxygen may be administered via several different methods. Table 6.5 provides an overview of equipment, oxygen flow rate, and the percentage of oxygen delivered.

Table 6.5

Oxygenation Equipment Overview		
Equipment	Flow Rate	FiO$_2$ Delivered
Nasal cannula	2–6 L/min	24%–50%
Simple face mask	5–10 L/min	35%–60%
Venture (Venti) face mask	10 L/min	Color-coded nozzles: Blue: 24% White: 28% Yellow: 35% Red: 40% Green: 60%
Non-rebreather mask	10 L/min	60%–80%

VENTILATOR MODES

Intubation and mechanical ventilation are employed when noninvasive measures are not effective. Respiratory failure evidenced by increasing CO_2, impending ventilatory failure, hypoxemia, or respiratory muscle fatigue is an indicator for intubation and mechanical ventilation. Various ventilator modes are available depending on the patient's pathophysiology. Refer to Appendix E: Respiratory and Ventilator Terminology for a comprehensive list of different ventilator modes. Close coordination and clear communication with the respiratory therapist are vital in planning the interdisciplinary care of the ventilated patient. The respiratory therapist is a crucial resource for troubleshooting, airway management, and safe care of the patient.

Fast Facts

All intubated patients should always have an Ambu bag connected to an oxygen flowmeter at the bedside. In the event of ventilator malfunction or power loss, disconnect the patient from the ventilator and provide manual respirations via the Ambu bag.

For an intubated patient who requires transport, always ensure a full tank of oxygen is connected to an Ambu bag.

SPECIAL INTERVENTIONS

- High-frequency ventilation (HFV) is a specialized type of ventilation that allows for very high respiratory rates, sometimes up to 900 breaths/min, with a low tidal volume. HFV is typically used for patients with specific pathophysiology such as ARDS. There are three types of HFV:

  1. High-frequency oscillatory ventilation (HFOV): Respiratory rate of up to 900 breaths/min with gas pushed into the lungs during inspiration and pulled out during expiration. Used for patients who remain hypoxic and are not responding to normal ventilator settings.
  2. High-frequency jet ventilation (HFJV): Respiratory rate of 100 to 200 breaths/min. Through a special endotracheal tube adaptor, a "jet" of gas flows into the airway at high pressure for a short duration.
  3. High-frequency positive pressure ventilation (HFPPV): With advancing technology, this setting is rarely used. Respiratory rate is usually 90 to 100 breaths/min with higher tidal volumes than HFOV or HFJV.

- ECMO: A form of cardiorespiratory bypass utilized in the critical care setting. By providing oxygenation and pulmonary support for patients with ARDS in lieu of traditional ventilator settings, it provides an opportunity for the lungs to rest and heal. ECMO may also be used as a bridge to lung transplant.

Resources

Diepenbrock, N. H. (2015). *Quick reference to critical care* (5th ed.). Philadelphia, PA: Wolters Kluwer.

Hinkle, J. L., & Cheever, K. H. (2017). *Brunner & Suddarth's handbook of laboratory and diagnostic tests* (3rd ed.). Philadelphia, PA: Wolters Kluwer.

Jones, J., & Fix, B. (2015). *Critical care notes: Clinical pocket guide* (2nd ed.). Philadelphia, PA: F.A. Davis.

Urden, L. D., Stacy, K. M., & Lough, M. E. (2016). *Priorities in critical care nursing* (7th ed.). St. Louis, MO: Elsevier.

References

American Association of Critical-Care Nurses. (2017). Oral care for acutely and critically ill patients. *Critical Care Nurse, 37*(3), e19–e21. doi:10.4037/ccn2017179. Retrieved from https://www.aacn.org/~/media/aacn-website/clincial-resources/practice-alerts/oralcarepractalert2017.pdf

Burns, S. M., & Delgado, S. A. (2019). *AACN essentials of critical care nursing* (4th ed.). New York, NY: McGraw-Hill.

Morton, P. G., & Fontaine, D. K. (2018). *Critical care nursing: A holistic approach* (11th ed.). Philadelphia, PA: Wolters Kluwer.

Urden, L. D., Stacy, K. M., & Lough, M. E. (2020). *Priorities in critical care nursing* (8th ed.). St. Louis, MO: Elsevier.

7

Cardiovascular Critical Care

The leading cause of mortality in the United States is cardio-vascular disease, with approximately 630,000 Americans dying from heart disease each year. In 2015, 366,000 died from coronary heart disease. An understanding of the predominant critical care admission diagnoses related to cardiovascular disease is crucial.

In this chapter, you will learn:

1. How to conduct a cardiovascular assessment
2. How to care for patients with specific cardiac conditions
3. Invasive hemodynamic monitoring
4. Various methods of cardiac support

CARDIAC ASSESSMENT

Completion of an in-depth cardiovascular assessment is an important aspect of caring for a patient in any critical/acute care setting. The major components of the cardiovascular assessment are:

1. Inspection of general appearance, including jugular venous distention and the apical impulse
2. Palpation of peripheral pulses, capillary refill, and edema
3. Auscultation of heart sounds
4. EKG interpretation
5. Vital signs

DIAGNOSES

The development of coronary artery disease (CAD) contributes to multiple cardiovascular system–related problems, leading to morbidity and mortality. The multiple risk factors that contribute to CAD are classified as modifiable or nonmodifiable. A general overview of these risk factors are listed in Table 7.1.

Acute Coronary Syndrome

The term "*acute coronary syndrome*" or ACS is used to describe several cardiac-related events, including unstable angina (USA), non-ST-elevated myocardial infarction (NSTEMI), and ST-elevated myocardial infarction (STEMI). (Refer to Appendix D: Basic EKG Rhythm Examples for EKG rhythms.)

- Stable angina: Chest pain that is predictable and caused by a similar pattern, activity, or event. Typically patients achieve pain control within 5 minutes of onset with rest and the use of sublingual nitroglycerin.
- USA: The result of limited or insufficient blood flow through the coronary artery. USA is a change in the previously established stable pattern of angina and requires medical intervention. Cardiac biomarkers are not elevated.
- NSTEMI: Partial blockage of a coronary artery producing ST-segment depression. Moderate damage may be caused to the left ventricle.

Table 7.1

Modifiable and Nonmodifiable Coronary Artery Disease Risk Factors	
Modifiable Risk Factors	**Nonmodifiable Risk Factors**
Blood pressure	Age
Cigarette/tobacco use	Gender
Serum cholesterol/lipid levels	Family history
Diet	Race
Lifestyle and physical activity	

Source: Adapted from National Institute of Health (nih.gov); Urden, L. D., Stacy, K. M., & Lough, M. E. (2020). *Priorities in critical care nursing* (8th ed.). St. Louis, MO: Elsevier

- STEMI: Total blockage of a coronary artery producing ST-segment elevation or new left bundle branch block (LBBB). Cardiac biomarkers are significantly elevated, and there is potential for major damage to the left ventricle. See Figure 7.1.

Fast Facts

Remember the acronym MONA for the initial steps in the treatment of a patient with ACS.

Morphine: Administer morphine for chest pain unrelieved by nitrates.

Oxygen: Oxygen via nasal cannula will provide more oxygen delivery to the myocardium.

Nitrates: Initially, start with sublingual nitroglycerin to dilate coronary vasculature.

Aspirin: Unless the patient is anaphylactically allergic, aspirin is proven to reduce morbidity and mortality in patients with ACS. If allergic, administer ticlopidine or clopidogrel.

Note: MONA is an acronym and not the actual sequence of interventions.

Causes

Coronary arteries may become blocked due to the rupture of a plaque, new thrombosis, or coronary artery spasm. Therefore, the flow of blood to the myocardium is limited or ceases.

Depending on what coronary artery is blocked, specific changes in the 12-lead EKG will be evident. Table 7.2 depicts the location of the infarct, associated EKG changes, coronary artery involvement, and signs and symptoms.

Signs and Symptoms

Patients with ACS present with the following symptoms:

- Midsternal chest pain, described as pressure, fullness, or squeezing of the chest
- Shortness of breath
- Nausea
- Diaphoresis
- Chest pain that radiates to the jaw, left arm, neck, or back

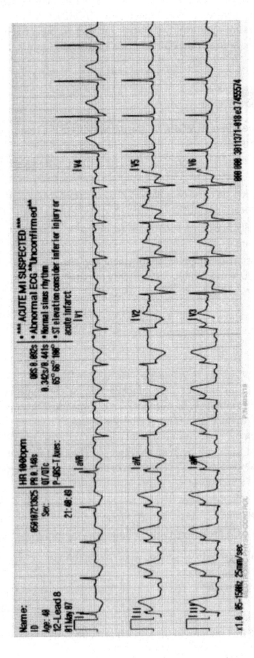

Figure 7.1 Suspected acute myocardial infarction.

Source: Buettner, J. R. (2017). *Fast facts for the ER nurse* (3rd ed.). New York, NY: Springer Publishing Company.

Table 7.2

Coronary Artery Occlusion and Myocardial Infarction

Coronary Artery	Myocardium	EKG Lead	Signs and Symptoms
Proximal left anterior descending	Anterior wall	V_1–V_4	Left ventricular pump failure Cardiogenic shock Death
Left main	Anterior wall	V_1–V_6, I, and aVL	Left ventricular pump failure Cardiogenic shock Death
Circumflex	Left lateral wall	I, aVL, V_5, and V_6	
Right coronary artery	Inferior wall	II, III, and aVF	Conduction disturbances Heart block Bradydysrhythmias

Source: Adapted from Burns, S. M., & Delgado, S. A. (2019). *AACN essentials of critical care nursing* (4th ed.). New York, NY: McGraw-Hill; Jones, J., & Fix, B. (2015). *Critical care notes: Clinical pocket guide* (2nd ed.). Philadelphia, PA: F.A. Davis; and Urden, L. D., Stacy, K. M., & Lough, M. E. (2020). *Priorities in critical care nursing* (8th ed.). St. Louis, MO: Elsevier.

Fast Facts

Lab Findings in Acute MI

	Increased Levels	Level Peaks	Remains Elevated
Creatine kinase-muscle/brain	3 to 8 hours after chest pain	12 to 24 hours	48 to 72 hours
Troponin	Within 3 to 12 hours after MI	14 to 48 hours	5 to 14 days

CK-MB, creatine kinase-muscle/brain.

Interventions

USA

- Medical treatment includes oxygen, nitroglycerin, and/or morphine for pain control, beta-blocker, antiplatelets, and heparin. Further diagnostic criteria as indicated.

NSTEMI

- In addition to treatment for USA, a diagnostic cardiac catheterization may be performed. During this procedure, if a coronary artery is significantly narrowed due to plaque, a coronary intervention will be performed, and a stent may be placed.

STEMI

- Fibrinolytics: Administer within 30 minutes of patient contact with the healthcare system (hospital or paramedic/emergency medical services). Fibrinolytics should be administered in settings where percutaneous transluminal coronary intervention (PTCA) is not feasible or readily available.
- Percutaneous coronary intervention (PCI), PTCA, and stenting: The process of inserting a catheter into the coronary artery and removing the blockage. A balloon catheter may open the blockage, while a stent is then placed to maintain the patency of the artery. For patients experiencing a STEMI, this process should be completed within 90 minutes of arrival at the hospital.
- Coronary artery bypass grafting (CABG): In the event of a failed PTCA, CABG is warranted on an emergency basis. Generally, the surgery is a scheduled event for a patient with multiple blocked coronary arteries or if there is major blockage of one of the major coronary arteries, such as the left main or right coronary artery. In the event of a failed PTCA, or inadvertent dissection of the coronary artery during PTCA, emergency CABG may need to be performed. Other indicators for emergency CABG are:
  - Recurrent ischemia
  - Ventricular septal wall or papillary muscle rupture
  - Cardiogenic shock occurring within 36 hours of myocardial infarction (MI), new LBBB with multivessel or left main CAD
  - Recurrent ventricular dysrhythmias with greater than 50% left main lesion or triple vessel disease

Heart Failure

A cardiac dysfunction in which the heart cannot pump enough blood to meet the body's needs. In hospitalized patients older than 65 years, it is the leading diagnosis. Heart failure is a progressive, nonreversible disease process. The progression of the disease is dependent on the cause and underlying structural abnormalities. Over time the disease will progress.

Causes

Heart failure may be caused by structural changes that impair the ability of the ventricles to either fill or eject blood. Structural changes may be caused by MI, valvular dysfunction, infection, cardiomyopathy, cardiotoxins, and uncontrolled hypertension.

Signs and Symptoms

Patient presentation is dependent on the extent of heart failure and the degree of ejection fraction. Patients with an ejection fraction of less than 40% will demonstrate the clinical signs and symptoms of heart failure. Further, signs and symptoms may vary if heart failure is isolated to the right or left side of the heart. The New York Heart Association (NYHA) Functional Classification of Heart Failure assigns patients into four groups. See Table 7.3.

Table 7.4 compares the differences between right-sided and left-sided heart failure.

Interventions

Patient care is based on relieving the symptoms, improving cardiac performance, and correcting the underlying cause. Frequently, the

Table 7.3

New York Heart Association Functional Classification of Heart Failure	
Class	Definition
I	Normal daily activity does not initiate symptoms
II	Normal daily activity initiates symptoms such as shortness of breath and fatigue, which subside with rest
III	Minimal activity initiates symptoms; usually symptom-free at rest
IV	Any type of activity will initiate symptoms; symptoms are present at rest

Source: Adapted from Dolgin, M., Fox, A. C., Gorlin, R., Levin, R. I., & Criteria Committee, New York Heart Association. (1994). *Nomenclature and criteria for diagnosis of diseases of the heart and great vessels* (9th ed.). Boston, MA: Lippincott Williams and Wilkins.
Original source: Criteria Committee, New York Heart Association, Inc. (1964). *Diseases of the heart and blood vessels. Nomenclature and criteria for diagnosis* (6th ed., p. 114). Boston: Little, Brown.

Table 7.4

Signs and Symptoms of Left-Sided and Right-Sided Heart Failure	
Left-Sided Heart Failure	**Right-Sided Heart Failure**
Dyspnea, shortness of breath	Right upper quadrant pain
PND	Peripheral edema
S_3 and S_4 gallop rhythm	Hepatomegaly and splenomegaly
Jugular venous distention	Jugular venous distention
Frothy, pink-tinged sputum/pulmonary edema	Ascites
Tachycardia	Pulmonary hypertension
Confusion and restlessness	Increased central venous pressure

PND, paroxysmal nocturnal dyspnea.

Source: Adapted from Burns, S. M., & Delgado, S. A. (2019). *AACN essentials of critical care nursing* (4th ed.). New York, NY: McGraw-Hill; Jones, J., & Fix, B. (2015). *Critical care notes: Clinical pocket guide* (2nd ed.). Philadelphia, PA: F.A. Davis; Urden, L. D., Stacy, K. M., & Lough, M. E. (2020). *Priorities in critical care nursing* (8th ed.). St. Louis, MO: Elsevier.

diagnosis of heart failure is made in the critical care unit when the patient is admitted with shortness of breath and pulmonary edema. After the patient is stabilized, diagnostic tests will be utilized to determine the underlying cause. These tests may include:

- Cardiac catheterization
- Echocardiography
- Diagnostic imaging

After the underlying cause is determined, a long-term treatment plan is formulated. If the cause is structural, such as a valvular abnormality, surgery may be indicated.

Fast Facts

Patient Education for Heart Failure

1. Pathophysiology of heart failure
2. Nutrition: Low salt diet; limit fluid intake
3. Fluid balance: Daily weight, monitoring fluid intake and output, peripheral edema, and signs of fluid overload

(continued)

(*continued*)

4. Shortness of breath: Increasing shortness of breath, sleeping upright or with several pillows, sleeping in a recliner should be reported to the healthcare professional
5. Activity: Planned activity and rest periods in order to conserve energy
6. Medications: Name of each medication, indication, when/ frequency to take, dosage, and side effects

Despite interventions and adherence to the treatment regimen, heart failure is a progressive disease without recovery or repair. Palliative care options should be discussed early in the disease process with the primary goal of symptom management.

Infections of the Heart

Endocarditis

Endocarditis is the infection or inflammation of the inner layers of the heart.

Causes: Generally caused by a bacterial infection and may affect the heart valves, chordae tendineae, septum, and the inner chambers of the heart.

Signs and Symptoms: Patients may present with flu-like symptoms, such as fever, chills, fatigue and weakness, nausea and vomiting, and headache. Additional signs specific to endocarditis will include:

- Chest pain
- Loud, regurgitant murmur
- Pericardial friction rub
- Petechiae on the conjunctiva, neck, chest, and abdomen

Interventions:

- Antibiotics as prescribed
- Cardiac support as indicated
- Avoid anticoagulants due to the risk of cerebral hemorrhage.

Pericarditis

Pericarditis is the inflammation of the outer layer of the heart leading to fluid accumulation within the pericardial sac.

Causes: May be an acute or chronic manifestation. Acute pericarditis is generally the result of a specific event such as an MI, surgery (CABG), or trauma. Chronic pericarditis may last for several months and be the result of autoimmune disease, radiation therapy, chemotherapeutic agents, or idiopathic.

Signs and Symptoms: Patient complaints may be related to the cause of the pericarditis. Generally, patients may complain of:

- Fever
- Dyspnea
- Orthopnea
- Cough
- Fatigue

Fast Facts

Pericarditis may present with complaints of chest pain. A classic presentation is the patient leaning forward while sitting to relieve pain. The complaint of pain increases while leaning back or lying down. Pain may be described as sharp, stabbing, or burning.

Interventions: Care for the patient with pericarditis is focused on relieving the pain and treating the cause. Generally, patients are treated with the following:

- Nonsteroidal anti-inflammatory agents
- Morphine for severe pain
- Antibiotics or antifungals if the pericarditis is the result of an infection
- Monitor for sign and symptoms of cardiac tamponade
- May require surgical intervention such as pericardiocentesis, pericardial window, or pericardiotomy

THERAPEUTIC HYPOTHERMIA

Also referred to as induced hypothermia or targeted temperature management (TTM). This therapy is initiated in certain patients after cardiac arrest to reduce the damage to the brain from a lack of blood and oxygen supply. The body's core temperature is reduced to between 32°C and 34°C and maintained for approximately 24 hours. Indications for therapeutic hypothermia include:

- Heart surgery
- Cerebral edema
- Ischemic cerebral or spinal injury
- Cardiac arrest with asystole, pulseless electrical activity (PEA), ventricular fibrillation, or ventricular tachycardia.

There are three phases of therapeutic hypothermia:

1. Induction
2. Maintenance
3. Rewarming

Refer to your institution's protocol for specific equipment use and patient criteria.

HEMODYNAMIC MONITORING

Arterial Line

An arterial line (A-line) is usually inserted into the patient's radial artery. A-lines are inserted in patients with unstable vital signs for blood pressure monitoring and for frequent lab tests, including arterial blood gas monitoring. Figure 7.2 depicts a normal arterial waveform pattern.

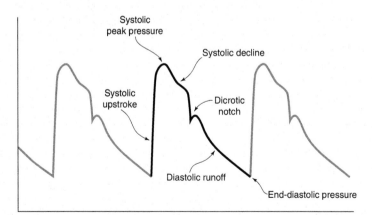

Figure 7.2 Normal arterial waveform.

Source: Yartsev, A. (2013–2019). *Normal arterial line waveforms.* Retrieved from https://derangedphysiology.com/main/cicm-primary-exam/required-reading/cardiovascular-system/Chapter%207.6.0/normal-arterial-line-waveforms

Fast Facts

Always perform an Allen's test prior to insertion of an A-line. The Allen's test determines if the patient's ulnar artery circulation is adequate to supply blood to the hand in the event the radial artery is occluded or has minimal circulation when the catheter is inserted.

1. Apply pressure to both the radial and ulnar arteries.
2. Watch for pallor of the hand.
3. Release pressure on the ulnar artery.
4. Color should return to the hand within 6 seconds.

Central Line and Central Venous Pressure

Central lines are generally inserted in the internal jugular vein or subclavian vein and advanced through the subclavian vein above the right atrium. Central lines may have multiple lumens designed to infuse large amounts of fluids, vasopressors, or blood products. One of the lumens may be used to determine the central venous pressure (CVP). This pressure is reflective of the patient's volume status. Normal CVP is 2 mmHg to 6 mmHg. Table 7.5 lists the causes of increased or decreased CVP.

Table 7.5

Causes of Increased or Decreased Central Venous Pressure (CVP)	
Increased CVP	**Decreased CVP**
Circulatory overload	Hemorrhage
Cardiac tamponade	Third spacing
Right ventricular failure	Extreme vasodilation (shock)
PEEP	
Severe mitral stenosis	
Pulmonary edema	
COPD	

COPD, chronic obstructive pulmonary disease; PEEP, positive end-expiratory pressure.

Source: Adapted from Burns, S. M., & Delgado, S. A. (2019). *AACN essentials of critical care nursing* (4th ed.). New York, NY: McGraw-Hill; Diepenbrock, N. H. (2015). *Quick reference to critical care* (5th ed.). Philadelphia, PA: Wolters Kluwer; Jones, J., & Fix, B. (2015). *Critical care notes: Clinical pocket guide* (2nd ed.). Philadelphia, PA: F.A. Davis; and Urden, L. D., Stacy, K. M., & Lough, M. E. (2020). *Priorities in critical care nursing* (8th ed.). St. Louis, MO: Elsevier.

Pulmonary Artery Catheter

The pulmonary artery (PA) catheter may be inserted through the internal jugular vein or subclavian vein and advanced through the right side of the heart and into the PA. The PA catheter is used to assess and monitor left ventricular function and determine cardiac output, preload, contractility, and afterload. The patient's hemodynamic profile may be calculated, and these numbers will guide fluid and vasopressor therapy. (Refer to Appendix B: Hemodynamic Parameters for normal parameters.)

CARDIOVASCULAR SUPPORT

Intra-Aortic Balloon Pump

This is used for temporary, mechanical circulatory support for patients in cardiogenic shock, postoperative support, and MI. Also known as counterpulsation, the intra-aortic balloon pump (IABP) is designed to increase blood and oxygen to the coronary arteries and myocardium. The device will increase preload and decrease afterload, thereby increasing cardiac output, decreasing myocardial oxygen consumption, and decreasing systemic vascular resistance.

A large catheter with a 30-mL balloon is inserted into the femoral artery and advanced to a specific point. The balloon will inflate during ventricular diastole and deflate just prior to ventricular systole, increasing the amount of blood in the ventricle during diastolic filling. Prior to systole, the balloon deflates, which decreases the impedance to ejection with an overall effect of increasing cardiac output. The coronary arteries receive their blood flow during ventricular diastole; therefore, the balloon pump enhances coronary artery blood flow.

Ventricular Assist Device

Offering more support than the IABP, a ventricular assist device (VAD) may be inserted for patients with end-stage cardiac disease, candidates awaiting a heart transplant, patients in cardiogenic shock after an MI, or patients who have undergone coronary pulmonary bypass. Devices used as a bridge to recovery include the Abiomed BVS 5000. The HeartMarte II VAD is commonly used as a bridge to transplant.

Smaller VADs may be placed in the cardiac catheterization lab following coronary intervention. An example of this is the Abiomed Impella. This device is inserted through the femoral artery and advanced through the aortic valve. By removing blood from the left ventricle and propelling it into the ascending aorta, the patient's cardiac output is enhanced.

Temporary Pacemaker

Temporary pacemakers may be initiated through a transcutaneous or transvenous approach.

- Transcutaneous pacemaker activity is provided through the external cardioverter/defibrillator.
- Transvenous pacemaker requires a lead wire to be inserted either through the brachial, internal or external jugular, subclavian or femoral vein and advanced to the heart. The lead is attached to an external pacemaker generator.

Whether a transcutaneous or transvenous pacemaker, the following settings must be programmed:

- Mode: Fixed/asynchronous or demand/synchronous
- Rate: Demand: set at 10 beats/min above the patient's rate; fixed: set at 70 to 100 beats/min
- Output (mA) or capture: Amount of voltage needed to stimulate the myocardium
- Sensitivity (mV) or millivolts: Determines when the pacemaker fires

Resources

Centers for Disease Control and Prevention. (n.d.). *Heart disease fact sheet.* https://www.cdc.gov/dhdsp/data_statistics/fact_sheets/fs_heart_disease .htm

Hinkle, J. L., & Cheever, K. H. (2017). *Brunner & Suddarth's handbook of laboratory and diagnostic tests* (3rd ed.). Philadelphia, PA: Wolters Kluwer.

Morton, P. G., & Fontaine, D. K. (2018). *Critical care nursing: A holistic approach* (11th ed.). Philadelphia, PA: Wolters Kluwer.

References

Burns, S. M., & Delgado, S. A. (2019). *AACN essentials of critical care nursing* (4th ed.). New York, NY: McGraw-Hill.

Diepenbrock, N. H. (2015). *Quick reference to critical care* (5th ed.). Philadelphia, PA: Wolters Kluwer.

Jones, J., & Fix, B. (2015). *Critical care notes: Clinical pocket guide* (2nd ed.). Philadelphia, PA: F.A. Davis.

Urden, L. D., Stacy, K. M., & Lough, M. E. (2020). *Priorities in critical care nursing* (8th ed.). St. Louis, MO: Elsevier.

8

Shock and Multiple-Organ Dysfunction Syndrome

Shock is generally defined as inadequate circulation to meet the demands of the body. The causes of shock vary from cardiac to hypovolemic to severe allergic reaction. Regardless of the cause, shock moves through progressive stages. Identifying the cause and intervening appropriately are crucial to prevent patient death.

In this chapter, you will learn:

1. The definition of shock
2. The stages of shock
3. Caring for patients in different shock states
4. The definition of multi-organ dysfunction syndrome (MODS)
5. Caring for patients with MODS

SHOCK

Patients admitted into the ICU may present with various forms and stages of shock. The shock may be the result of an "inadequate pump," as in cardiogenic shock when the heart is unable to pump enough volume, or "insufficient volume in the tank" as in hypovolemic shock. Another classification of shock is distributive that may be attributed to sepsis, anaphylaxis, or neurogenic. Shock syndrome moves through four stages:

1. Initial: Decreased cardiac output
2. Compensatory: As the body senses a decrease in cardiac output, the heart rate increases, and the venoarterial bed constricts, shunting blood to the vital organs in an attempt to increase the cardiac output
3. Progressive: Metabolism changes from aerobic to anaerobic. Anaerobic metabolism results in large amounts of lactic acid production, leading to lactic acidosis
4. Refractory: The shock is unresponsive to interventions and the process is irreversible

TYPES OF SHOCK

Hypovolemic

This is a result of a decreased circulating volume of blood, or intravascular volume. This type of shock, sometimes referred to as an "empty tank," means there is not enough circulating blood volume in the body.

Causes

May be caused by hemorrhage, burn, dehydration, ascites, or acute pancreatitis. In some cases, such as burns, fluids within the intravascular space move to the interstitial spaces, resulting in decreased intravascular circulating volume.

Signs and Symptoms

Signs and symptoms are related to the amount of volume that is lost. Table 8.1 provides an outline of the stages of shock, volume loss, and patient signs and symptoms.

Interventions

Interventions are aimed at correcting the underlying cause and replacing the lost circulating volume with crystalloids, colloids, blood products, or a combination of fluids.

Cardiogenic

This is caused by the failure of the heart to pump enough blood due to loss of myocardial contractility. In cardiogenic shock, the engine malfunctions.

Table 8.1

Stages of Shock

Shock Stage	Volume Loss	Patient Signs and Symptoms
Class I Mild/initial stage	Up to 15%, or 750 mL	Symptom-free or mild anxiety
Class II Mild to moderate/ compensatory stage	15%–30%, or 750–1,500 mL	Increased heart rate, narrowed pulse pressure, increased respiratory rate, decreased urine output, skin is cool and pale, jugular veins appear flat
Class III Moderate to severe/ progressive stage	30%–40%, or 1,500–2,000 mL	Blood pressure begins to decrease, and the heart rate may increase to 120 beats/min, oliguria, skin is cool, ashen, and clammy. The patient may be confused as the result of decreased cerebral perfusion
Class IV Severe/refractory stage	>40%, or 2,000 mL	Severe tachycardia and dysrhythmias, hypotension, skin is cyanotic, mottled and diaphoretic, urine output ceases, and organ failure ensues. The patient becomes unresponsive

Causes

Acute myocardial infarction with loss of 40% or more of the myocardium is the most common cause.

Signs and Symptoms

Decreased cardiac output triggers compensatory mechanisms, resulting in tachycardia; systolic blood pressure (SBP) less than 90 mmHg; decreased urine output; cool, clammy skin; and a weak, thready pulse.

Interventions

Increase the contractility of the myocardium through positive inotropic agents such as dobutamine and dopamine. Decrease the preload and afterload through mechanical support with an intra-aortic balloon pump (IABP).

DISTRIBUTIVE SHOCK STATES

Neurogenic

Occurring predominantly in patients with spinal cord injuries above the level of T6, neurogenic shock is the result of severe autonomic dysfunction. The dysfunction may last several days to several months, requiring pressor agents during the acute phase.

Causes

Injury to the sympathetic pathways of the nervous system will result in loss of vasomotor tone and sympathetic innervation to the heart, depending on the location of the spinal cord injury. Loss of vasomotor tone will result in:

- Profound hypotension due to massive vasodilation
- Bradycardia
- Decreased cardiac output
- Decreased heart rate along with hypotension
- Hypothermia caused by heat loss through vasodilation

Signs and Symptoms

The patient demonstrates hypotension, bradycardia, and decreased central venous pressure (CVP). The patient's skin may feel warm instead of cold and clammy like in the case of other types of shock due to the extensive vasodilation.

Interventions

Focus on raising the blood pressure (BP) through fluid resuscitation or the use of vasopressors, causing vasoconstriction. Maintain an SBP greater than 90 mmHg. Vasopressors may consist of both alpha-adrenergic agonists, such as norepinephrine, that result in vasoconstriction, and beta-adrenergic agonists, such as dopamine, that increase the heart rate. Maintain the patient's body temperature with warming measures, such as warm blankets and commercial warming devices.

Anaphylactic

A hypersensitive reaction or severe allergic reaction caused by an antibody–antigen response. This response releases histamine and causes systemic reactions, including wheezing, laryngeal edema, bronchospasm, pulmonary edema, tachycardia, vasodilation, and ultimately shock. Immediate intervention may be required to prevent complete cardiovascular collapse and death.

Causes

Anaphylactic shock may be the result of medications, such as penicillin, chemotherapy agents, immunotherapy, foods, and venom from insect bites.

Signs and Symptoms

Signs and symptoms begin to develop immediately after exposure to the noxious agent. Symptoms initially start with cutaneous reactions, such as urticaria, erythema, and angioedema. Next, respiratory symptoms develop, including wheezing, stridor, or hoarseness, and the patient may complain of a feeling of fullness or lump in the throat. Bronchoconstriction will restrict gas exchange, leading to hypoxia. Massive vasodilation from the antigen–antibody reaction will result in hypotension, reflex tachycardia, and decreased cardiac output.

Interventions

Administer epinephrine as soon as signs and symptoms develop. Based on the patient's status, prepare for rapid sequence intubation.

Fast Facts

Epinephrine is the first-line treatment for anaphylactic shock. The dose is as follows:

- 0.2 to 0.5 mg of a 1:1,000 solution IM given in the anterolateral thigh. Repeat every 5 to 15 minutes.
- 0.05 to 0.1 mg of a 1:10,000 solution IV for severe hypotension, given over 5 minutes.
- A continuous infusion of epinephrine may be initiated.

Rapid fluid replacement may require 1L of fluid given over 5 to 10 minutes.

In addition to fluid volume resuscitation and epinephrine, the following medications may be used, depending on patient response:

- Diphenhydramine (Benadryl): 1 to 2 mg/kg via slow IV injection
- Ranitidine: 1 mL/kg IV over 10 to 15 minutes
- Inhaled beta-adrenergic treatments for bronchospasm
- Corticosteroids to help prevent a delayed reaction

Septic

Severe sepsis and septic shock are the leading causes of hospital mortality with more than 1 million hospitalizations annually.

Causes

Invading microorganisms may either be gram-negative or gram-positive bacteria, fungi, and viruses. The microorganisms may invade the body through the respiratory tract, urinary tract, wounds, the gastrointestinal system, or implanted medical devices.

Signs and Symptoms

Signs and symptoms depend on the stage of the sepsis cascade. The sequence of events leading to septic shock are:

1. Clinical insult: Initial exposure and response to the microorganism
2. Systemic inflammatory response (SIRS): A generalized systemic reaction to the invading organism characterized by the manifestation of at least two of the following:
   a. Temperature greater than 38°C or less than 36°C
   b. Heart rate greater than 90
   c. Respiratory rate greater than 20
   d. White blood cells (WBC) greater than 12,000/mm³ or less than 4,000/mm³ with more than 10% bands
3. Sepsis: Documentation of the progression to SIRS and a positive infection
4. Severe sepsis: Organ dysfunction along with hypoperfusion or hypotension. This may be evidenced by:
   a. Altered mental state
   b. Lactate greater than 4 mmol/L
   c. Urine output less than 0.5 mL/kg/hr for more than 2 hours
   d. Acute lung injury
   e. Platelet count less than 100,000 µL
5. Septic shock: Persistent hypotension despite fluid resuscitation and inadequate tissue perfusion

Interventions

The Surviving Sepsis Campaign (SSC) outlines guidelines for the management of severe sepsis and septic shock. This "bundle" of care consists of evidence-based practice guidelines to be performed within the first 3 and 6 hours. Table 8.2 outlines the SSC bundles.

Therapy goals:

- MAP: >65 mmHg
- CVP: 8 to 12 mmHg

Table 8.2

Surviving Sepsis Bundles: Evidence-Based Practice Guidelines for Managing Severe Sepsis and Septic Shock

Complete within the first 3 hours:	Complete within 6 hours:
1. Fluid resuscitation with 30 mL/kg of crystalloid for hypotension or lactate ≤4 mmol/L	1. Maintain MAP ≤65 mmHg with vasopressors if unresponsive to fluid boluses
2. Obtain blood cultures: aerobic and anaerobic	2. Goal CVP is ≤8 mmHg
3. Administer broad spectrum antibiotics within 1 hour	3. Measure central venous oxygen saturation with the goal of ≤70%
4. Obtain serum lactate level	4. Remeasure lactate if initial level elevated

CVP, central venous pressure; MAP, mean arterial pressure.

Source: Adapted from AACN Bold Voices; www.survivingsepsis.org

- Central venous oxygen saturation ($S_{cv}O_2$): 65%
- Urine output: >0.5 mL/kg/hr
- Lactate level within normal limits

Multi-Organ Dysfunction Syndrome

A failure of two or more organ systems, generally starting with the lungs followed by the kidneys and heart.

Causes

Patients at great risk for MODS may have the following diagnoses:

- Sepsis
- Multiple trauma
- Shock states
- Acute pancreatitis
- Multiple blood transfusions
- Inadequate fluid resuscitation

Signs and Symptoms

Patients experiencing these diagnoses may progress to pulmonary failure followed rapidly by a failure of the kidneys and heart. The signs and symptoms include severe hypotension, decreasing oxygen saturation, or the inability to maintain satisfactory oxygen saturation with pulmonary support, decreased urine output, and a Glasgow Coma Scale (GCS) of <15.

Interventions

There is no specific intervention for MODS. Supportive care includes vasopressors to maintain an adequate BP, fluid resuscitation, intubation and ventilation, and continuous renal replacement therapy; however, none of these interventions have demonstrated an improved survival rate. Mortality rate is directly related to the number of failing organ systems.

Fast Facts

Nurses play a key role in preventing infections and recognizing the early signs of sepsis.

Prevention includes:

1. Hand hygiene
2. Implementing measures to prevent ventilator-acquired pneumonia (VAP)
3. Invasive catheter care following hospital protocols and guidelines
4. Wound care
5. Monitoring patients for systemic inflammatory response syndrome (SIRS) and following hospital notification guidelines

Resources

American Association of Critical-Care Nurses. (2019). Two strategies succeeding against sepsis. *AACN Bold Voices, 11*(1), 10.

Barbar, S. D., Clere-Jehl, R., Bourredjem, A., Hernu, R., Montini, F., Bruyère, R., . . . IDEAL-ICU Trial Investigators and the CRICS TRIGGERSEP Network. (2018). Timing of renal-replacement therapy in patients with acute kidney injury and sepsis. *New England Journal of Medicine, 379*(15), 1431–1442. doi:10.1056/NEJMoa1803213

Burns, S. M., & Delgado, S. A. (2019). *AACN essentials of critical care nursing* (4th ed.). New York, NY: McGraw-Hill.

Diepenbrock, N. H. (2015). *Quick reference to critical care* (5th ed.). Philadelphia, PA: Wolters Kluwer.

Hinkle, J. L., & Cheever, K. H. (2017). *Brunner & Suddarth's handbook of laboratory and diagnostic tests* (3rd ed.). Philadelphia, PA: Wolters Kluwer.

Jones, J., & Fix, B. (2015). *Critical care notes: Clinical pocket guide* (2nd ed.). Philadelphia, PA: F.A. Davis.

Morton, P. G., & Fontaine, D. K. (2018). *Critical care nursing: A holistic approach* (11th ed.). Philadelphia, PA: Wolters Kluwer.

Society of Critical Care Medicine. (n.d.). Retrieved from http://www.survivingsepsis.org/Pages/default.aspx

Urden, L. D., Stacy, K. M., & Lough, M. E. (2020). *Priorities in critical care nursing* (8th ed.). St. Louis, MO: Elsevier.

9

Gastrointestinal Critical Care

The most common gastrointestinal (GI)-related admissions into critical care are for acute bleeding episodes. GI bleeding may be upper or lower, with upper GI (UGI) bleeding carrying a higher mortality rate of 6% to 15%. Lower GI (LGI) bleeding has a mortality rate of 5% and generally resolves spontaneously. Other common admissions are for patients experiencing acute pancreatitis and hepatic encephalopathy.

In this chapter, you will learn:

1. How to conduct a GI assessment
2. How to care for patients with specific GI conditions
3. How to initiate enteral feedings in the ICU

GASTROINTESTINAL ASSESSMENT

A focused GI assessment follows a specific pattern:

1. Inspection
2. Auscultation
3. Percussion
4. Palpation

GASTROINTESTINAL BLEED

GI bleeding is described as upper or lower, with UGI bleeding occurring four times more frequently than lower. The anatomical landmark, the ligament of Treitz, determines if the bleed is upper or lower. Patient care is planned based on the location and cause of the bleeding.

UGI Bleed

Acute bleeding occurring proximal to the ligament of Treitz is defined as UGI bleeding. It can be classified as variceal or nonvariceal.

Causes

The most common causes of UGI bleeding are:

1. Peptic ulcer disease: Gastric and duodenal ulcers
2. Esophageal varices: Increased portal vein pressure causing rupture of esophageal or gastric varices
3. Mallory–Weiss tear: A tear of the gastric mucosa along the gastroesophageal junction; frequently found in alcoholic patients from intense vomiting associated with binge drinking
4. Stress-related erosive syndrome: Occurs frequently in hospitalized patients; sudden onset, minimal bleeding, and self-limiting syndrome
5. Esophagitis/gastritis: Many causes, but mainly related to nonsteroidal anti-inflammatory drug (NSAID) use, steroids, alcohol abuse, and severe stress
6. Neoplasm: Cancers occurring in the stomach or esophagus

Signs and Symptoms

One sign of UGI bleeding is hematemesis that is bright red, brown, or coffee-ground in color. Based on the amount of blood loss, the patient will display signs and symptoms associated with hypovolemic shock:

1. Tachycardia
2. Hypotension
3. Pale, cool, clammy skin
4. Decreased urine output

Interventions

1. Initiate fluid resuscitation with a large-bore IV needle at two sites administering crystalloids, colloids, and blood products, as directed.

2. Insert nasogastric tube (NG) for decompression of gastric contents and lavage.
3. Begin preparation for endoscopic procedures to determine the cause of bleeding and interventions to stop or control the bleeding. If the bleeding is caused by varices, sclerotherapy will be implemented with injection therapy into the variceal.

Fast Facts

Pharmacological Therapy for UGI Bleeding

1. Antacids
2. Histamine blockers: Cimetidine, ranitidine, famotidine
3. Cytoprotective agents: Sucralfate
4. Proton-pump inhibitors (PPI): Omeprazole, esomeprazole, lansoprazole
5. IV medication: Pantoprazole
6. Mucosal barrier enhancers: Colloidal bismuth, prostaglandins

LGI Bleed

LGI bleeding occurs distal to the ileocecal valve and may originate from the colon, rectum, and anus.

Causes

The most common causes of LGI bleeding are:

1. Diverticulosis: This is the most common cause of LGI bleeding requiring ICU admission. (Diverticula are small, sac-like protrusions in the colon wall. These are prone to rupture that may result in either massive bleeding requiring intervention or bleeding that spontaneously ceases.)
2. Neoplasm: Cancers of the lower intestinal tract
3. Inflammatory bowel disease
4. Trauma: Penetrating or severe blunt force trauma resulting in intestinal bleeding
5. Ischemia: Occlusion of the intestinal tract due to obstruction

Signs and Symptoms

The presence of melena (dark, tarry stools) or hematochezia (maroon stools or bright-red blood from the rectum) is a sign of LGI bleeding. If bleeding is due to diverticulitis, the patient will report a painless, sudden onset of maroon-colored stools. Based on the amount of blood loss, the patient may present with signs and symptoms consistent with hypovolemia.

Interventions

Fluid resuscitation is needed as indicated by the patient's vital signs. Rule out UGI bleeding by inserting an NG tube. If bleeding is localized to the LGI region, prepare for a colonoscopy.

Acute Pancreatitis

Acute pancreatitis is an inflammation of the pancreas with autodigestion from exocrine enzymes produced by the pancreas. Severity may range from mild/self-limiting to necrotizing pancreatitis. The mortality rate is related to the severity of the inflammation, with necrotizing pancreatitis carrying a 30% mortality rate. Severe pancreatitis may lead to SIRS and multi-organ dysfunction syndrome (MODS).

Causes

Idiopathic pancreatitis accounts for 10% to 20% of the diagnoses. Other triggers of acute pancreatitis include:

1. Alcohol abuse
2. Infection such as mumps
3. Gallstones and biliary tract disease
4. Blunt abdominal trauma
5. Various medications, including glucocorticoids, NSAIDs, furosemide, angiotensin-converting enzyme (ACE) inhibitors, and estrogen

Signs and Symptoms

Severe knife-like pain along the mid-epigastric or mid-abdominal region that may radiate to the back. Additional signs and symptoms include:

1. Nausea and vomiting
2. Abdominal distention
3. Rebound tenderness
4. Fever
5. Tachypnea and tachycardia
6. Signs associated with hypovolemia from vomiting and third spacing

Interventions

Aggressive fluid resuscitation and electrolyte replacement is prescribed. Manage pain with analgesics and positioning in the knee-chest position. Insert the NG tube for vomiting or obstruction. Monitor for MODS.

Fast Facts

The choice of analgesics depends on the patient's response. There are no evidence-based studies demonstrating the use of meperidine as superior to other analgesics such as morphine and fentanyl. Careful administration and assessment of the patient's response should guide the choice of pain control medications.

Hepatic Encephalopathy

Hepatic encephalopathy is associated with severe liver dysfunction and the inability of the liver to process and remove ammonia in the bloodstream. The accumulating ammonia level has a toxic effect on the brain.

Causes

Acute liver failure may lead to hepatic encephalopathy.

Signs and Symptoms

Signs and symptoms are dependent on the extent of the acute liver failure. Table 9.1 outlines the staging of hepatic encephalopathy and associated signs and symptoms.

Table 9.1

Stages of Hepatic Encephalopathy

Staging	Hepatic Encephalopathy
Stage I	Marked by either euphoria or depression, mild confusion, impaired mentation, normal EEG
Stage II	Lethargy, moderate confusion, marked asterixis, abnormal EEG
Stage III	Marked confusion, sleeping but arousable, incoherent speech, abnormal EEG
Stage IV	Coma, unresponsive to noxious stimuli, asterixis absent, abnormal EEG

Source: Adapted from Morton, P. G., & Fontaine, D. K. (2018). *Critical care nursing: A holistic approach* (11th ed.). Philadelphia, PA: Wolters Kluwer; Urden, L. D., Stacy, K. M., & Lough, M. E. (2020). *Priorities in critical care nursing* (8th ed.). St. Louis, MO: Elsevier; Burns, S. M., & Delgado, S. A. (2019). *AACN essentials of critical care nursing* (4th ed.). New York, NY: McGraw-Hill.

Interventions

Interventions are focused on reducing the ammonia level in the blood. Care includes:

1. Administration of oral neomycin. It alters the intestinal flora so the blood is not broken down and converted to ammonia.
2. Administration of lactulose orally, by NG tube, or by retention enema. Lactulose produces an acidic environment that will draw ammonia out of the blood and excrete it through a laxative effect.
3. Monitoring of electrolytes.
4. Restriction of dietary proteins.

Fast Facts

Avoid lactated Ringer's IV solution as the lactate is converted to lactic acid and more ammonia is produced.

Enteral Nutrition

Do not overlook nutritional intake in critically ill patients. Early enteral feedings are crucial to prevent malnutrition, which may place patients at greater risk for morbidity and mortality, poor surgical outcomes, and increased ventilator days. The Joint Commission requires all patients to undergo a nutritional screening, and critical care patients are no exception. Based on the screening results, initiate plans for enteral feedings. Current evidence suggests that nurse-driven protocols may provide for quicker placement on a nutritional supplement, increased feedings as tolerated with increased caloric intake.

Patients who are unable to tolerate enteral feedings or whose diagnoses prevent enteral feedings should be placed on parenteral nutrition. Patients on parenteral nutrition are at higher risk of infectious complications and must be carefully monitored with the parenteral nutrition discontinued as soon as possible and the patient transitioned to enteral feedings.

Fast Facts

Nutritional recommendations:
25 cal/kg/day based on the patient's ideal weight.
1.2–1.5 g/kg/day of protein.
For severely malnourished patients, maintain caloric intake at
15–20 kcal/kg to minimize electrolyte shifts.

Resources

Diepenbrock, N. H. (2015). *Quick reference to critical care* (5th ed.). Philadelphia, PA: Wolters Kluwer.

Gibson, W., Scaturo, N., & Allen, C. (2018). Acute management of upper gastrointestinal bleeding. *Advanced Critical Care, 29*(4), 369–376. doi:10 .4037/aacnacc2018644

Hinkle, J. L., & Cheever, K. H. (2017). *Brunner & Suddarth's handbook of laboratory and diagnostic tests* (3rd ed.). Philadelphia, PA: Wolters Kluwer.

Jones, J., & Fix, B. (2015). *Critical care notes: Clinical pocket guide* (2nd ed.). Philadelphia, PA: F.A. Davis.

Orinovsky, I., & Raizman, E. (2018). Improvement of nutritional intake in intensive care unit patients via nurse-led enteral nutrition feeding protocol. *Critical Care Nurse, 38*(3), 38–45. doi:10.4037/ccn2018433

References

Burns, S. M., & Delgado, S. A. (2019). *AACN essentials of critical care nursing* (4th ed.). New York, NY: McGraw-Hill.

Morton, P. G., & Fontaine, D. K. (2018). *Critical care nursing: A holistic approach* (11th ed.). Philadelphia, PA: Wolters Kluwer.

Urden, L. D., Stacy, K. M., & Lough, M. E. (2020). *Priorities in critical care nursing* (8th ed.). St. Louis, MO: Elsevier.

10

Renal Critical Care

Acute kidney injury (AKI), previously termed acute renal failure (ARF), is commonly seen in critical care patients. The mortality rate of critical care patients with AKI is 15% to 60%. It is essential that the critical care nurse differentiates between prerenal, intrarenal, and postrenal failure in order to assess, intervene, and evaluate the patient's response to the care plan. Monitoring fluid and electrolyte balance is a vital function to prevent further deterioration. Specific interventions to support patients with AKI are common in critical care and include continuous renal replacement therapy (CRRT).

In this chapter, you will learn:

1. How to conduct a renal assessment
2. The definiton and decription of AKI
3. How to care for patients with specific kidney injury
4. How to implement CRRT

RENAL ASSESSMENT

Renal assessment includes a careful history and physical examination and review of current laboratory results. The history will reveal factors that may contribute to altered renal function and exposure to medications or toxins that can impair kidney function. The patient may report an unexplained weight gain of greater than 2 pounds over a period of 1 to 2 days.

The physical exam assesses for peripheral edema and bleeding along the flank area as a result of trauma. Specific lab results to monitor include blood urea nitrogen (BUN) and creatinine. An increase in BUN indicates a deterioration in kidney function. Similarly, an increase in creatinine is further indicative of kidney injury. The ratio of BUN to creatinine may be an indicator of the level of AKI—prerenal, intrarenal, or postrenal. Electrolytes excreted by the kidney need to be carefully monitored. In renal failure, potassium may not be excreted, and increased potassium levels may affect the conduction system of the heart, leading to dysrhythmias.

Relying on urine output to determine kidney function may be problematic as the use of diuretics may increase urine output but not change the course of kidney disease. Monitoring BUN, creatinine, and glomerular filtration rate (GFR) is the best determinant of kidney function.

ACUTE KIDNEY INJURY

Fast Facts

The acronym RIFLE may be used to determine a critically ill patient's risk of developing AKI. RIFLE stands for:

Risk
Injury
Failure
Loss
End-stage kidney disease
R, I, and F are increasing stages of severity. L and E are the outcome criteria.

Prerenal Kidney Injury

This is the most common cause of AKI.

Causes

AKI is caused by decreased perfusion of the kidneys as a result of hypovolemia, hypotension, or cardiogenic or septic shock. A decrease in blood flow to the kidneys results in a reduced GFR leading to azotemia—an increase in creatinine and urea in the bloodstream.

Signs and Symptoms

Signs and symptoms include decreased urine output of less than 400 mL/24 hours, increased serum urea (BUN) and creatinine, edema, jugular venous distention, and electrolyte imbalances—that is, increased potassium and sodium—as well as tachycardia with dysrhythmias.

Fast Facts

BUN:Creatinine Ratio

Normal BUN to creatinine ratio is 10:1. The ratio is a good indicator of the AKI level.

- In intrarenal kidney failure, the ratio of 10:1 remains the same even with elevated BUN and creatinine levels.

In prerenal kidney failure, the ratio is greater than 10:1.

Interventions

Correcting the underlying cause is the primary treatment. Reversal of prerenal kidney injury has a high success rate if treated within the first 24 hours of onset. Interventions are focused on correcting fluid volume, hypotension, and reversing shock states. If not treated and reversed, prerenal kidney injury will progress to acute tubular necrosis (ATN).

Intrarenal Kidney Injury

Causes

This is caused by injuries and various disease states that lead to hypoperfusion of the glomerular apparatus, leading to a decrease in the GFR. Injuries include burns and crush injuries; disease processes include infections, lupus erythematosus, malignant hypertension, and diabetes mellitus. Regardless of the cause, prolonged hypoperfusion of the kidney leads to nonreversible damage and ATN. The three phases of AKI related to intrarenal impairment are outlined in Table 10.1.

Interventions

Patient care in AKI is dependent on the phase of the disease process. The plan of care is focused on:

- Fluid/volume balance
- Monitoring and treating electrolyte imbalances

Table 10.1

Phases of Acute Kidney Injury

Phase	Characteristics	Complications	Length of Duration
Oliguric	↑ BUN ↑ Creatinine ↓ Urine output	Fluid overload Hyperkalemia (K⁺)	Few days to several weeks
Diuretic—gradual return of renal function	↑ BUN ↑ Creatinine ↑ Urine output	May excrete up to 5 L/d Electrolyte imbalances Fluid deficit	7–10 d
Recovery	Stabilization of lab results	Some degree of renal insufficiency is common	3–12 mon

BUN, blood urea nitrogen.

Source: Adapted from Burns, S. M., & Delgado, S. A. (2019). *AACN essentials of critical care nursing* (4th ed.). New York, NY: McGraw-Hill; Morton, P. G., & Fontaine, D. K. (2018). *Critical care nursing: A holistic approach* (11th ed.). Philadelphia, PA: Wolters Kluwer; Urden, L. D., Stacy, K. M., & Lough, M. E. (2020). *Priorities in critical care nursing* (8th ed.). St. Louis, MO: Elsevier.

- Treating metabolic acidosis
- Maintaining adequate nutrition
- Preventing additional kidney damage
- Managing CRRT

Postrenal Kidney Injury

This is not a common cause of renal injury in the critical care patient. Increased pressure in the kidneys results in a decrease in the GFR.

Causes

This is caused by obstructions blocking the flow of urine beyond the kidney, such as tumors, stenosis of the ureter or urethra, renal calculi, enlarged prostate, and kinked urinary catheter.

Signs and Symptoms

Sudden, abrupt cessation of urine flow.

Interventions

Removal of the obstruction.

Rhabdomyolosis

This is the increased release of creatine and myoglobin from damaged muscle cells. If treated early with crystalloid fluids, the mortality rate is low. Myoglobin in large quantities may occlude the kidneys, reducing the GRF.

Causes

Damage may occur from trauma, heat exhaustion/stroke, status epilepticus, burns, illegal drug use (cocaine), or other events, leading to severe muscle breakdown.

Signs and Symptoms

Signs and symptoms are related to the event that caused muscle cell damage. Close monitoring of creatine kinase levels reveals the amount of myoglobin and correlated kidney damage.

Interventions

Fluid resuscitation with crystalloids is the primary treatment plan. Carefully monitor serum potassium levels as increased levels may occur from the breakdown of cells releasing intracellular potassium into the bloodstream. This may lead to life-threatening dysrhythmias.

Nephrotoxic Injury From Contrast Media

Causes

The use of IV radiopaque contrast or "dye" during radiologic studies may cause kidney injury and AKI.

Signs and Symptoms

Signs and symptoms include and increase in serum creatinine of 0.5 mg/dL or more or a 25% increase from the patient's baseline value within 3 days of the radiologic tests.

Interventions

Aggressively hydrate with IV normal saline solution during and after the procedure. Discontinue the use of some nephrotoxic medications prior to the procedure; specifically, the medication Metformin is stopped the day before the procedure and then held for 2 days post procedure.

TREATMENT MODALITIES FOR RENAL FAILURE

Continuous Renal Replacement Therapy

Different from hemodialysis (HD), which is episodic, CRRT is done over a period of time for 24 hours/day. Similar to HD, it removes fluid and the buildup of toxins from the blood through ultrafiltration.

CRRT is tolerated in patients who are hemodynamically unstable and unable to tolerate the higher flow rate of HD. CRRT is dependent on the patient's status and may be provided through different modalities:

- Continuous arteriovenous hemofiltration (CAVH) requires an arteriovenous (AV) site. It functions similarly to slow continuous ultrafiltration (SCUF). Replacement fluid is used, and mean arterial pressure (MAP) must be at least 60 mmHg.
- Continuous venovenous hemofiltration (CVVH) requires a blood pump, removes fluid via ultrafiltration and solutes via convection. Replacement fluid is given either before or after filtration.
- Continuous arteriovenous hemodialysis (CAVHD) is a combination of CAVH and HD. Aided by a pump, dialysate flows in the opposite direction of the blood, allowing diffusion and convection to occur. Fluid and molecules are removed with this method.
- Continuous venovenous hemodialysis (CVVHD) requires a dual-lumen venovenous access site and involves ultrafiltration, diffusion, and osmosis. No replacement fluid is needed. Blood flow is 10 to 180 mL/min.
- SCUF requires arteriovenous access and is often used for removing large amounts of fluid. Blood flow is 10 to 180 mL/min.
- Continuous venovenous hemodiafiltration (CVVHDF) requires a dual-lumen venovenous access site, blood pump, and dialysate. Replacement fluid is necessary and is capable of moving high volumes of fluid hourly.

CRRT is provided and monitored by a specially trained ICU registered nurse, which is different from HD that is provided and monitored by the HD nurse. Venous access is initiated by the physician and is typically placed in the jugular or subclavian vein.

Femoral access is only used if no other access is feasible. Femoral sites are avoided due to increased risk of infection and impaired mobility.

CRRT requires a specific blood pump that is different from a standard HD machine. The filter must be changed every 24 to 48 hours per hospital policy.

Hemodialysis

Used in patients who are hemodynamically stable during AKI, HD lasts for 3 to 4 hours/day and may be done daily. Patients in chronic renal failure receive HD on an outpatient basis three or four times per week. Patients who are hemodynamically unstable will not tolerate conventional HD because it involves the movement of approximately 300 mL of blood at any given time, along with major shifts in fluid and electrolytes.

HD may be utilized for patients with drug overdose or exposure to certain toxins such as bromide, chloral hydrate, ethanol, ethylene glycol, lithium, methanol, or salicylate. In these situations, HD should be initiated within 4 to 6 hours of exposure.

Similar to CRRT, central vascular access is obtained, and blood is moved through an external dialyzer and then returned to the body. The dialyzer contains a semipermeable membrane that filters out toxins, waste, metabolic by-products, and excess fluid.

Fast Facts

Medications that can be cleared through dialysis:

Acetaminophen	Bretylium
Aminoglycosides	Cephalosporins
Aspirin	Cimetidine
Atenolol	Esmolol
Aztreonam	Nipride
Angiotensin-converting enzyme inhibitors	Most penicillins
	Ranitidine

Resources

Diepenbrock, N. H. (2015). *Quick reference to critical care* (5th ed.). Philadelphia, PA: Wolters Kluwer.

Dirkes, S. M. (2016). Acute kidney injury vs. acute renal failure. *Critical Care Nurse, 36*(6), 75–76. doi:10.4037/ccn2016170

Hinkle, J. L., & Cheever, K. H. (2017). *Brunner & Suddarth's handbook of laboratory and diagnostic tests* (3rd ed.). Philadelphia, PA: Wolters Kluwer.

Jones, J., & Fix, B. (2015). *Critical care notes: Clinical pocket guide* (2nd ed.). Philadelphia, PA: F.A. Davis.

Thompson, A., Li, F., & Gross, A.K. (2017). Considerations for medication management and anticoagulation during continuous renal replacement therapy. *AACN Advanced Critical Care, 28*(1), 51–63 doi:10.4037/aacnacc2017386

References

Burns, S. M., & Delgado, S. A. (2019). *AACN essentials of critical care nursing* (4th ed.). New York, NY: McGraw-Hill.

Morton, P. G., & Fontaine, D. K. (2018). *Critical care nursing: A holistic approach* (11th ed.). Philadelphia, PA: Wolters Kluwer.

Urden, L. D., Stacy, K. M., & Lough, M. E. (2020). *Priorities in critical care nursing* (8th ed.). St. Louis, MO: Elsevier.

11

Endocrine Critical Care

The most common endocrine abnormalities in critical care involve blood glucose control. Diabetic patients may be admitted with diabetic ketoacidosis (DKA) or hyperglycemic hyperosmolar state with dangerously high blood glucose levels. Diabetic patients who are typically within control may require higher dosages of insulin due to the body's stress response to the illness. Monitoring blood glucose, fluid status, and electrolyte balance is key to patient care. Other common endocrine disease states encountered in the critical care unit include diabetes insipidus (DI), syndrome of inappropriate antidiuretic hormone (SIADH), acute adrenal crisis, and myxedema coma.

In this chapter, you will learn:

1. How to care for patients with specific endocrine disorders
2. Glucose control in critically ill patients

DIAGNOSES

Diabetic Ketoacidosis

DKA is defined as hyperglycemia with acidosis. It is most common in type 1 diabetics and may manifest in type 2 diabetics. An absence or inadequate amount of insulin results in severe hyperglycemia, dehydration, and electrolyte abnormalities.

Causes

The most common causes of DKA are infection, newly diagnosed diabetes, and missed insulin doses. Other less common causes include trauma, myocardial infarction, pancreatitis, and stroke.

Signs and Symptoms

DKA is characterized by three abnormalities:

1. Hyperglycemia
2. Ketonemia
3. Metabolic acidosis with a large anion gap

Further, DKA may be classified as mild, moderate, and severe. See Table 11.1.

Patients presenting with mild DKA may be alert and responsive, whereas patients with moderate DKA exhibit increased drowsiness. Patients in severe DKA states will be in a coma.

Other signs and symptoms include:

- Polyuria and polydipsia
- Anorexia, nausea, and vomiting
- Abdominal pain and cramping
- Weight loss
- Hypothermia
- Tachypnea
- Hypotension
- Tachycardia and shock
- Dehydration

Table 11.1

Classifications of Diabetic Ketoacidosis			
	Mild	Moderate	Severe
Glucose	>300 mg/dL	>300 mg/dL	>300 mg/dL
Bicarbonate	15–18 mEq/L	10–14 mEq/L	<10 mEq/L
pH	<7.30	<7.20	<7.1

Source: Adapted from Burns, S. M., & Delgado, S. A. (2019). *AACN essentials of critical care nursing* (4th ed.). New York, NY: McGraw-Hill; Morton, P. G., & Fontaine, D. K. (2018). *Critical care nursing: A holistic approach* (11th ed.). Philadelphia, PA: Wolters Kluwer; Urden, L. D., Stacy, K. M., & Lough, M. E. (2020). *Priorities in critical care nursing* (8th ed.). St. Louis, MO: Elsevier

Interventions

Treatment focuses on correcting dehydration, replacing insulin, reversing ketoacidosis, and replenishing electrolytes.

1. Correcting dehydration: Patients with DKA may lose 5% to 10% of their body weight in fluids. Correctly assessing the hydration status and commencing fluid replacement is crucial to prevent circulatory collapse. One liter of normal saline (0.9%) is infused immediately, with further fluid replacement guided by lab results and the patient's hemodynamic status. It is not uncommon to administer over 6 L of fluid.

2. Replace insulin: In moderate-to-severe DKA, give an IV bolus of regular insulin, usually at a dose of 0.1 units/kg, followed by a continuous insulin infusion of 0.1 units/kg/h. Insulin infusion is titrated to the patient's glucose levels. Monitor glucose levels every hour.

3. Reverse ketoacidosis: Ketoacidosis begins to reverse by fluid management and insulin administration.

4. Replenish electrolytes: Potassium replacement is guided by serum potassium levels and renal function.
   a. For $K^+ < 3.3$ MEq/L, hold insulin; KCl 20 to 30 mEq/h until >3.3
   b. For $K^+ > 5.2$ mEq/L, begin insulin; hold KCl; check K^+ level every 2 hours

Fast Facts

Current Research

A study by Compton, Ahlborn, and Weidehoff (2017) demonstrated that a RN–directed blood glucose protocol did not increase nursing workload. Their research provided evidence that the number of hypoglycemic incidents were reduced and patients maintained an adequate glycemic control.

Hyperosmolar Hyperglycemic State

Hyperosmolar hyperglycemic state (HHS) is a hyperglycemic state common in type 2 diabetics. Unlike DKA, an acidotic state does not occur in HHS. Blood glucose is extremely high in HHS, usually greater than 600 mg/dL. This highly elevated blood glucose level results in serum hyperosmolality, leading to osmotic diuresis, which in turn results in major dehydration. As type 2 diabetics generally have confounding comorbidities, the mortality rate for HHS ranges from 5% to 20%.

Causes

The primary cause of HHS in a type 2 diabetic is an infection, usually pneumonia or urinary tract infection. Although patients take oral agents for type 2 diabetes, it becomes unstable due to the infection. Other causes of HHS include:

- Stroke
- Myocardial infarction
- Trauma
- Major surgery
- Stress of a critical illness

HHS may evolve over several days or weeks.

Signs and Symptoms

The patient may report a history of several days of blurred vision, malaise, polyuria, polydipsia, weight loss, and weakness. By the time the patient seeks medical care, dehydration may be so severe that the patient presents with confusion, seizure, and coma. Other signs and symptoms include:

- Severe hyperglycemia with blood glucose >600 mg/dL
- Tachycardia
- Hypotension
- Tachypnea
- Serum hyperosmolarity >320 mOsm/kg
- Absent or insignificant ketoacidosis

Interventions

The initial intervention focuses on fluid resuscitation. Fluid deficit may be as great as 150 mL/kg of body weight.

1. Correct dehydration: Normal saline is infused at a rate of 1 L/h while monitoring blood pressure (BP) and central venous pressure (CVP). Several liters may be required to achieve a normal BP and CVP. The serum sodium level is closely monitored and determines the need for 0.9% normal saline or 0.45% saline.
2. Insulin replacement: Fluid resuscitation corrects hyperglycemia; however, insulin is administered to prevent acidosis and facilitate the cellular uptake of glucose. Initial dose may be 0.15 units/kg IV bolus, followed by a continuous infusion. Glucose levels are monitored hourly.

3. Replenish electrolytes: Monitoring the potassium level guides replacement. Similar to DKA, if the serum potassium level is <3.3 mEq/L, insulin is held until potassium is replaced.

Is it DKA or HHS? Table 11.2 compares and contrasts the differences and similarities between DKA and HHS.

Fast Facts

Insulin will drive potassium into the cell. Therefore, for DKA and HHS patients with a serum potassium level less than 3.3 mEq/L, potassium must be replaced before insulin is administered. If this is not done, the hypokalemic state will worsen, leading to the possibility of lethal cardiac dysrhythmias.

Remember: Potassium before glucose!

Table 11.2

Characteristics of Diabetic Ketoacidosis (DKA) Versus Hyperosmolar Hyperglycemic State (HHS)		
	DKA	**HHS**
History of diabetes mellitus	Type 1	Type 2
Onset	Rapid	Slow
Respiratory rate	Hyperventilation	Slightly rapid
Breath odor	Acetone or sweet	None
Blood glucose elevation	Elevated	Markedly elevated
Serum sodium	Mild hyponatremia	Hypernatremia
Serum ketones	Positive	Negative
Serum potassium	Hyperkalemia initially, then hypokalemia	Within normal limits
Serum osmolality	Slightly elevated	Markedly elevated
Acidosis	Metabolic acidosis	Negative

Source: Adapted from Burns, S. M., & Delgado, S. A. (2019). *AACN essentials of critical care nursing* (4th ed.). New York, NY: McGraw-Hill; Morton, P. G., & Fontaine, D. K. (2018). *Critical care nursing: A holistic approach* (11th ed.). Philadelphia, PA: Wolters Kluwer; Urden, L. D., Stacy, K. M., & Lough, M. E. (2020). *Priorities in critical care nursing* (8th ed.). St. Louis, MO: Elsevier

Syndrome of Inappropriate Antidiuretic Hormone

Increased and sustained release of antidiuretic hormone (ADH) from the posterior pituitary gland results in the kidneys reabsorbing water, leading to dilutional hyponatremia. The classic presentation of SIADH is hypotonic hyponatremia (serum sodium less than 125 mEq/L) with an elevated serum osmolality.

Causes

Although the pituitary gland produces and regulates ADH, the most common cause of SIADH is exogenous, implying that ADH is secreted from a different location. Most commonly, it is the result of a bronchogenic or pancreatic carcinoma. These tumors can independently secrete ADH. Other causes may include:

- Head injuries
- Pneumonia and lung abscess
- Central nervous system infection or tumors
- Medications: Antipsychotics, cytotoxic agents, nicotine, illicit substances
- Other endocrine disorders

Signs and Symptoms

The most common signs and symptoms include:

- Personality changes
- Headache
- Change in mental status
- Lethargy
- Abdominal cramps
- Decreased tendon reflexes
- Nausea, vomiting, anorexia
- Seizures
- Coma

Frequently, signs and symptoms are not exhibited until the serum sodium level is less than 125 mEq/L.

Interventions

Care of patients with SIADH focuses on three interventions:

1. Treating the underlying cause
2. Managing excessive water retention
3. Providing safe care for patients with a diminished level of consciousness

The underlying cause may or may not be treatable depending on the location and type of carcinoma. There are no medications that will completely suppress the release of ADH.

First, restrict fluids. In mild cases, this is sufficient. Patients with severe symptoms and acute hyponatremia require an infusion of 3% hypertonic saline solution and furosemide. Infusion of 3% saline must be carefully monitored and administered at a rate of 0.1 mg/kg/min to prevent volume overload and pulmonary edema. Usually, a total of 300 to 500 mL over 4 to 6 hours is sufficient to reverse the hyponatremia. The goal is to increase the serum sodium level by 1 to 2 mEq/h. Osmotic demyelination may occur if serum sodium is increased too rapidly, leading to severe neurologic damage or death. This neurologic damage is called "locked-in" syndrome. The patient is unable to speak or initiate any voluntary muscle movement other than the eyes. However, the patient is fully aware, can think, and feel.

Diabetes Insipidus

In contrast to SIADH, DI is an absolute or relative deficiency of ADH, termed central DI, or an insensitivity to the effects of ADH on the tubules, termed nephrogenic DI.

Causes

The causes of DI fall into two categories:

1. Vasopressin deficiency: The pituitary gland is unable to secrete ADH due to either tumors, vascular accidents (stroke or infarction of the area), infection, or neurosurgery.
2. Nephrogenic: Due to a genetic defect (inherited), the kidneys are unable to absorb water.

Patients with head trauma or those who underwent neurosurgery are closely monitored for DI for up to 7 to 10 days after the injury or surgery. DI may not manifest for at least 48 to 72 hours after the incident.

Signs and Symptoms

Regardless of the cause, patients with DI have the following signs and symptoms:

- Polydipsia
- Polyuria
- Increased serum osmolality
- Increased serum sodium

- Decreased urine osmolality
- Decreased urine specific gravity

Interventions

Goals of patient care include preventing dehydration and electrolyte imbalance. A hypotonic solution of 0.45% saline is rapidly infused to match urine output and prevent hypovolemic shock.

The most commonly used medication is desmopressin acetate (DDAVP), a synthetic ADH. DDAVP may be given intravenously, subcutaneously, or as a nasal spray. Unlike vasopressin (Pitressin), DDAVP is preferred due to minimal effect on patient's BP.

Adrenal Crisis (Addison's Disease)

Also known as acute adrenal insufficiency, adrenal crisis is the inability of the adrenal cortex to secrete aldosterone and cortisol, leading to hypoglycemia and hypovolemic shock.

Causes

The vast majority of cases are idiopathic (70%). Other precipitating causes of adrenal crisis include:

- Discontinuation of long-term corticosteroid therapy
- Sepsis
- Infection or injury to the adrenal gland
- Bilateral adrenalectomy
- Chronic adrenal insufficiency
- Medications
  - Suppression of the adrenal hormones
  - Enhanced steroid metabolism

Signs and Symptoms

Patients with adrenal insufficiency will demonstrate the following signs and symptoms:

- Hypoglycemia
- Fever
- Dehydration
- Hypotension
- Hypovolemic shock
- Electrolyte imbalance
- Severe muscle weakness and fatigue
- Nausea, vomiting, anorexia, diarrhea
- Altered mental status: Lethargy and confusion
- Unresponsive to vasopressors

Interventions

Adrenal insufficiency may lead to Addisonian crisis, which is a life-threatening condition. Interventions include fluid volume and electrolyte replacement and IV administration of corticosteroids. Carefully monitor and evaluate the patient's response to fluid and electrolyte replacement by assessing respiratory and cardiovascular function, BP, heart rhythm, skin color and temperature, and CVP.

Fast Facts

Never give insulin to a patient with Addison's disease. The resulting hypoglycemia may be fatal.

Myxedema Coma

The inability or deficiency of the thyroid gland to secrete an adequate amount of hormones to meet the metabolic demands of the body. Hypothyroidism may be primary or secondary. Primary hypothyroidism is a disorder of the thyroid gland. Secondary hypothyroidism may be caused by pituitary gland dysfunction, hypothalamic disorders, or peripheral resistance to thyroid hormones.

Causes

A variety of triggers may cause the life-threatening event of myxedema coma. The most common cause is pulmonary infection, trauma, stress, medications, and surgery. Other causes include:

- Thyroid gland destruction or dysfunction due to surgery, radioactive iodine, or external radiation to the neck
- Thyroiditis
- Medications: Amiodarone, lithium, iodides
- Thyroid-releasing hormone deficiency
- Thyroid stimulating hormone deficiency
- Infiltrative diseases: Sarcoidosis, lymphoma
- Autoimmune disease: Hashimoto's disease, post-Graves' disease

Signs and Symptoms

Hypothyroidism results in fatigue, weakness, anorexia, weight gain, decreased bowel sounds, and EKG changes. Myxedema coma is a rare complication of hypothyroidism. Patients may present with the following signs and symptoms:

- Severe depression
- Hypothermia: Body temperature as low as 80°, without shivering

- Hypoventilation
- Hypoxemia
- Hypotension
- Bradycardia
- Hypoglycemia

Interventions

Myxedema coma is a life-threatening condition and must be treated with a multisystem approach. For severe hypoventilation and hypoxemia, intubation and mechanical ventilation is indicated. IV infusions of hypertonic normal saline and glucose solutions support hypotension and hypoglycemia. For severe hypotension, IV vasopressors may be required. Hormone replacement occurs gradually to prevent sudden increase in metabolic function. For patients experiencing hypothermia, gradual rewarming is implemented with warm blankets.

GLUCOSE MANAGEMENT IN CRITICAL CARE PATIENTS

Patients in the ICU are under multiple sources of stress. For type 1 and type 2 diabetic patients whose blood glucose is generally under control, the stress response of disease, trauma, surgery, and shock may lead to hyperglycemia. Hyperglycemia may also develop in patients without a history of diabetes. A landmark research study in 2001 demonstrated a significant reduction in morbidity and mortality among critical care patients when blood glucose was tightly controlled between 80 and 110 mg/dL.

Specific conditions predisposing patients to hyperglycemia include:

- Sepsis
- Myocardial infarction
- Pregnancy
- Vasopressors such as norepinephrine, dopamine, dobutamine
- Liver failure
- Renal failure

Recommended serum glucose level in critically ill patients:

- 140 to 180 mg/dL
- Begin insulin IV drip for persistent glucose >180 mg/dL
- IV insulin is preferred to subcutaneous injections. Refer to your hospital-specific protocol.

Resources

Compton, F., Ahlborn, R., & Weidehoff, T. (2017). Nurse-directed blood glucose management in a medical intensive care unit. *Critical Care Nurse, 37*(3), 30–40. doi:10.4037/ccn2017922

Diepenbrock, N. H. (2015). *Quick reference to critical care* (5th ed.). Philadelphia, PA: Wolters Kluwer.

Finfer, S., Chittock, D. R., Su, S. Y., Blair, D., Foster, D., Dhingra, V., . . . Ronco, J. J. (2009). Intensive versus conventional glucose control in critically ill patients. *New England Journal of Medicine, 360*(13), 1283–1297. doi:10.1056/NEJMoa0810625

Hinkle, J. L., & Cheever, K. H. (2017). *Brunner & Suddarth's handbook of laboratory and diagnostic tests* (3rd ed.). (2018). Philadelphia, PA: Wolters Kluwer.

Jones, J., & Fix, B. (2015). *Critical care notes: Clinical pocket guide* (2nd ed.). Philadelphia, PA: F.A. Davis.

Van den Berghe, G., Wilmer, A., Hermans, G., Meersseman, W., Wouters, P. J., Milants, I., . . . Bouillon, R. (2006). Intensive insulin therapy in the medical ICU. *New England Journal of Medicine, 354*(5), 449–461. doi:10.1056/NEJMoa052521

Van den Berghe, G., Wouters, P., Weekers, F., Verwaest, C., Bruyninckx, F., Schetz, M., . . . Bouillon, R. (2001). Intensive insulin therapy in critically ill patients. *New England Journal of Medicine, 345*(19), 1359–1367. doi:10.1056/NEJMoa011300

Woodruff, D. W. (2016). *Critical care nursing made incredibly easy* (4th ed.). Philadelphia, PA: Wolters Kluwer.

References

Burns, S. M., & Delgado, S. A. (2019). *AACN essentials of critical care nursing* (4th ed.). New York, NY: McGraw-Hill.

Morton, P. G., & Fontaine, D. K. (2018). *Critical care nursing: A holistic approach* (11th ed.). Philadelphia, PA: Wolters Kluwer.

Urden, L. D., Stacy, K. M., & Lough, M. E. (2020). *Priorities in critical care nursing* (8th ed.). St. Louis, MO: Elsevier.

12

Trauma Critical Care

As the leading cause of death for all age groups less than 44 years, trauma costs the United States hundreds of billions of dollars each year. Instead of the term "accident," motor vehicle crash (MVC) and unintentional injury constitute the current terminology. Domestic violence, now termed intimate partner violence (IPV), is a leading cause of injury to women. Approximately 30% of all ICU admissions are for traumatic injuries. This chapter provides an overview of blunt and penetrating trauma leading to injury of the brain, thorax, abdomen, and musculoskeletal system.

Trauma patients are stabilized in the ED and may require surgery before being admitted to the critical care unit.

In this chapter, you will learn:

1. The care of patients experiencing various forms of trauma
2. A general approach to all trauma patients
3. Various mechanisms of trauma

TRAUMA

Blunt Trauma

Blunt trauma is most frequently seen with MVC, contact sports, falls, or blunt force injuries from fighting or use of an object such as a baseball bat. The injury occurs due to a sudden and rapid change in velocity, such as deceleration in a vehicle.

Fast Facts

Intimate Partner Violence

The Joint Commission now requires all patients to be screened for IPV during the health history assessment. Research has demonstrated that this screening is effective to identify women who are victims or who are in violent relationships.

MVC: Acceleration and Deceleration Injuries

The most common cause of blunt trauma is a motor vehicle crash. Prior to the crash, the occupant and the vehicle travel at the same speed. When the crash occurs, the occupant and the vehicle decelerate to zero, but not at the same rate. The occupant's body impacts with the car's interior, and the internal organs impact the body structures and surfaces within the body. Consequently, major vessels stretch and possibly tear as a result of the rapid deceleration.

Penetrating Trauma

These are injuries that penetrate the body and are caused by firearms, stabbing, or impalement, all of which damage the internal organs. The extent of internal injury relates to the size of the firearm and ammunition. Penetrating injuries may be high velocity or low velocity. The velocity of the injury determines the extent of tissue damage and cavitation. For example, shotguns are short-range, low-velocity weapons. Handguns and rifles are long-range, high-velocity weapons. Each of these produces penetrating injuries with varying degrees of internal damage.

Stab wounds relate to the type and length of the object and the angle of penetration. Stab wounds or impalement are a low-velocity injury. The extent of damage is determined by the length, width, and trajectory of the penetration and the presence of vital organs.

Thoracic Trauma

Trauma to the chest may be the result of blunt or penetrating injuries. Injuries may include the chest wall, lungs, heart, great vessels, and esophagus.

Causes

Blunt thoracic injury is usually the result of an MVC or fall. Penetrating injuries are directly related to the type of weapon, for example, high- or low-velocity missiles (handgun, rifle, shotgun) or knife. The following is an overview of thoracic traumatic injuries.

Thoracic Injuries

- Rib fracture: Rib fracture may be life-threatening when three or more ribs are fractured. Fracture of the first or second ribs requires a high degree of force and may result in injury to intrathoracic vasculature. Fracture to the middle ribs may result in lung injury and pneumothorax. Fractures of the seventh to 12th ribs may result in abdominal injuries to the spleen or liver.
- Flail chest: Caused by blunt trauma, flail chest is the fracture of a rib or ribs in two places resulting in a free-floating segment of rib. This causes a paradoxical movement of the chest wall.
- Ruptured diaphragm: Due to subtle and nonspecific symptoms, a ruptured diaphragm is often overlooked on initial assessment. Compressive trauma to the abdomen results in a tear or rupture of the diaphragm, with the possibility of abdominal contents herniating into the chest cavity.
- Tension pneumothorax: It is a perforation of the chest wall or pleural space that allows air to enter the pleural cavity during inspiration and become trapped. Pressure increases as more air enters the pleural space resulting in compression of the lung until it collapses. This is a life-threatening condition, and the pressure must be relieved as soon as possible.
- Open pneumothorax: Also known as a "sucking chest wound," an open pneumothorax is the result of a penetrating injury. An open pneumothorax is similar to a tension pneumothorax. The chest wall opening must be covered with an occlusive dressing such as a petroleum gauze until a chest tube is inserted or surgical intervention.
- Hemothorax: Bleeding into the pleural space results in a hemothorax. The bleeding may be from an artery, heart, or the great vessels. Arterial bleeding usually requires immediate surgical intervention. Low-pressure bleeding from the lung parenchyma is usually self-limiting, and the bleeding stops spontaneously.

Heart and Vascular Injuries

- Penetrating cardiac injuries: Injuries to the heart from penetrating objects such as missiles (bullets), stabbing, or impalement carries a very high mortality rate. Most deaths occur within minutes from exsanguination or tamponade.

- Cardiac tamponade: It refers to fluid accumulation within the pericardial sac causing increased pressure on the ventricles and atria, leading to decreased cardiac output and cardiogenic shock. Pericardiocentesis or surgical intervention is required to remove the fluid and relieve the pressure on the heart.
- Blunt cardiac injury: This injury is usually caused by MVC and direct force on the chest. The heart can be thrown again the chest wall or forced back against the thoracic vertebrae. Other injuries may be from being hit with a baseball or kicked by an animal.
- Aortic injury: Blunt aortic injuries (BAI) occur in less than 1% of MVCs but are lethal. BAI should be suspected if there is a fracture of the first or second rib, high sternal fracture, or left clavicular fracture.

Interventions

Care for the patient with chest trauma is individualized and depends on the type and extent of damage. Key interventions include:

- Airway support for oxygenation, ventilation, and cardiovascular status
- Monitoring of chest tube drainage and function
- Pain control
- Early mobility
- Prevention of complications
- Nutritional support

Abdominal Trauma

Abdominal injuries may be caused by blunt or penetrating trauma. The third leading cause of traumatic death, abdominal injuries are associated with multitrauma events. Hemorrhage and hollow organ perforation are life-threatening.

Causes

Blunt abdominal injuries usually result from MVCs, falls, and assaults. Abdominal trauma is more likely when a vehicle is struck from the side. Penetrating abdominal injuries are usually from gunshot wounds and stabbings. The following is an overview of abdominal traumatic injuries:

- Liver injuries: The liver may be injured by blunt or penetrating trauma. Nonoperative management is standard for patients who are hemodynamically stable. Continuously monitor the patient's response to therapy. Patients who remain unstable may require an exploratory laparotomy.

- Hollow viscus organs: These include the stomach, small intestine, and large intestine. Intestinal contents leak into the peritoneum resulting in peritonitis. Serial white blood cell count helps determine if hollow viscus injury (HVI) is present, which requires surgical intervention and repair.
- Spleen: Similar to liver injuries, the patient is monitored while being aggressively managed in the critical care unit. Hemodynamically unstable patients require surgery and a possible splenectomy to control bleeding.
- Kidneys: Blunt abdominal trauma may result in kidney injury. Gross hematuria may be present but is not always reflective of the extent of injury. The hematuria may clear within a few hours. Minor injury to the kidney is treated with observation. More severe injuries such as a devascularized segment of the kidney require surgery.

Fast Facts

Careful assessment and reassessment must occur in patients with suspected abdominal blunt trauma. Death is more likely to occur from abdominal blunt trauma than penetrating trauma.

Interventions

Care of the patient with abdominal trauma focuses on observation and assessment. Key interventions include:

- Monitoring for bleeding
- Infection prevention
- Nutritional support

Musculoskeletal Trauma

Musculoskeletal injuries include fractures, dislocation, and amputation. Generally, assessment of the musculoskeletal system after a traumatic injury is part of the secondary assessment as these injuries are generally not life-threatening. Complications from musculoskeletal injuries include compartment syndrome, deep vein thrombosis (DVT), pulmonary embolus (PE), and fat embolism syndrome. The following is an overview of musculoskeletal injuries:

- Fracture: Bone fractures are classified based on the type of fracture and if the injury is "closed" or "open." Closed fractures do not cause any breakage of the skin or protrudion of the bone segments. Care of the patient with a fracture depends on the type of fracture.

- Dislocation: Refers to the disruption of the articulating surfaces of a joint causing restricted mobility. Depending on the location, the force exerted that caused the dislocation, and the extent of the injury, vascular and nerve damage may occur.

- Amputation: Amputation from a cut or "guillotine" type of injury results in clean lines with well-defined edges, whereas a crush amputation results in more soft tissue damage.

- Pelvic fractures: Generally occurring from an MVC, pelvic fractures may be life-threatening as a result of acute blood loss.

Musculoskeletal injury complications include:

- Compartment syndrome: Traumatic injury to large muscles from fractures or crush injuries may result in tissue swelling and edema leading to compartment syndrome. Continued tissue swelling in a specific muscle compartment may lead to a lack of perfusion, ischemia, and nerve damage. The patient may complain of decreased sensation in the area, which is the most reliable early sign of compartment syndrome. Pressure within the muscle compartment may be measured using a specialized needle. Treatment is with a fasciotomy or a surgical opening of the skin and fascia to relieve pressure.

- DVT: All trauma patients are at risk of a DVT, especially those with musculoskeletal injuries. DVT prophylactic measures should be implemented on all trauma patients, including administration of low-dose heparin or low-molecular-weight heparin and the use of intermittent pneumatic compression devices. Refer to your institution's protocols.

- PE: Occurs when a blood clot dislodges and travels to the pulmonary artery. It is frequently seen in patients with a coexisting DVT. Signs and symptoms depend on the size of the embolus and the location within the pulmonary vasculature where it lodges. (Refer to Chapter 6, Respiratory Critical Care, for specific information on PEs.)

Traumatic Brain Injury

MVC, falls, and assaults comprise 80% of traumatic brain injury (TBI) admissions. TBI may be classified as:

- Acceleration injuries: When a moving object hits the head such as a baseball bat or missile (gunshot).

- Acceleration/deceleration injuries: When the head is in motion and strikes a stationary object such as an MVC, fall, or physical assault.
- Coup contrecoup injuries: These occur when the brain moves back and forth in the skull resulting in damage to both sides of the brain. This can result from MVC and falls.
- Rotational forces injuries: These occur when the brain twists within the skull causing stretching and tearing of blood vessels and neurons.
- Penetration injuries from missiles (bullets), shrapnel, or stabbings.

TBIs have a primary and secondary component. Primary injury occurs as a direct result of trauma to the brain. Secondary injury occurs due to cerebral edema, ischemia, and biochemical changes that occur in the brain as a result of the primary injury.

Interventions

Care of the patient with TBI focuses on controlling intracranial pressure (ICP) and promoting cerebral perfusion. Specific interventions include:

- Monitor and control ICP: Refer to Chapter 5, Neurological Critical Care, for details on ICP.
- Maintain cerebral perfusion: Cerebral perfusion pressure (CPP) between 50 and 70 mmHg.
- Prevent and treat seizures: Antiseizure medications should be given in the first 7 days of the injury. Seizures are associated with increased ICP and cerebral metabolic demands. Phenytoin is the recommended antiseizure medication during the acute period.
- Maintain a normal body temperature: Hyperthermia causes increased cerebrometabolic demands and may worsen secondary brain injury.
- Identify and manage sympathetic storming: Sympathetic storming is also known as paroxysmal sympathetic hyperactivity and is characterized by diaphoresis, agitation, flexion or extension posturing, restlessness, hyperventilation, tachycardia, and fever. Triggers include stressful events, loud noises such as alarms, and fever.
- Monitor fluid and electrolyte status: Carefully monitor intake and output as well as electrolyte status. Osmotic diuretics, commonly prescribed in brain injury patients, may cause dehydration and electrolyte imbalance. Monitor for signs of syndrome of inappropriate antidiuretic hormone (SIADH) or diabetes insipidus in the brain injured patient.

- Manage cardiovascular complications: Monitor cardiac function with EKG, cardiac enzyme levels, and echocardiography. Implement DVT prophylaxis according to hospital protocols.
- Manage pulmonary complications: Patients with TBI are at risk of acute lung failure, pneumonia, neurogenic pulmonary edema, and PE.
- Manage nutrition and maintain glycemic control: Brain injury may place the patient in a hypermetabolic and hypercatabolic state. Provide nutritional support as ordered and maintain tight glucose control.
- Manage musculoskeletal complications: Collaborate with physical therapy and occupational therapy for early mobility and interventions for an unresponsive patient. Preventing pressure ulcers and contractures ensures the patient is in the best physical condition for rehabilitation.
- Care for the family: Families of TBI patients need specific, consistent, and truthful information. Families need to be actively involved in patient care.

Resources

Burns, S. M., & Delgado, S. A. (2019). *AACN essentials of critical care nursing* (4th ed.). New York, NY: McGraw-Hill.

Diepenbrock, N. H. (2015). *Quick reference to critical care* (5th ed.). Philadelphia, PA: Wolters Kluwer.

Hinkle, J. L., & Cheever, K. H. (2017). *Brunner & Suddarth's handbook of laboratory and diagnostic tests* (3rd ed.). Philadelphia, PA: Wolters Kluwer.

Jones, J., & Fix, B. (2015). *Critical care notes: Clinical pocket guide* (2nd ed.). Philadelphia, PA: F.A. Davis.

Morton, P. G., & Fontaine, D. K. (2018). *Critical care nursing: A holistic approach* (11th ed.). Philadelphia, PA: Wolters Kluwer.

Urden, L. D., Stacy, K. M., & Lough, M. E. (2016). *Priorities in critical care nursing* (7th ed.). St. Louis, MO: Elsevier.

13

Transplant Critical Care

Currently, there are over 110,000 candidates on the organ transplant waiting list. The vast majority of these candidates are awaiting a kidney transplant (>94,000). In 2018, the most frequently transplanted organ was the kidney (21,167), followed by the liver (8,250) and the heart (3,408).

This chapter reviews the general guidelines for the care of a patient undergoing an organ transplant.

In this chapter, you will learn:

1. Specific disease states that may necessitate an organ transplant
2. Guidelines specific to kidney, liver, and heart transplants
3. General guidelines for the recovery of organ transplant recipients
4. The signs, symptoms, and potential treatment of transplant rejection

KIDNEY TRANSPLANT

Common reasons for a kidney transplant:

- Glomerular disease
  - Systemic lupus erythematosus
  - Sickle cell anemia
  - Amyloidosis
- Diabetes
  - Type 1 and type 2
- Polycystic kidneys

Kidney Transplant Guidelines

- Uncomplicated cases may go from the recovery room directly to the floor.
- Assess for pain over the transplant site and/or thick, yellow drainage from the incision. Both may indicate a urine leak.
- Anticipate renal ultrasounds on postoperative day 1.
- Complete bedrest without hip flexion on the side of the graft for 48 to 72 hours post-op.

Fast Facts

Acute kidney rejection occurs within the first postoperative week. Signs and symptoms specific to renal transplant rejection include elevated creatinine and increased blood urea nitrogen (BUN). Complications specific to kidney transplants include lymphocele development, thrombosis, ureteral obstruction, and the development of a urine leak.

LIVER TRANSPLANT

A liver transplant may involve the entire liver or sections/segments of the liver. Common conditions requiring a liver transplant include:

- Noncholestatic cirrhosis
- Biliary atresia
- Acute hepatic necrosis

Liver Transplant Guidelines

1. Monitor prothrombin time, partial thromboplastin time, fibrinogen, and factor V levels as ordered.
2. Monitor blood pressure; hypertension is common.
3. GI assessment: Monitor for ascites, bowel sounds, tenderness, nausea, vomiting and distention.
4. Do not reposition or irrigate the nasogastric tube without orders.
5. Measure abdominal girth every 12 hours.
6. Monitor liver function lab results as ordered.
7. Monitor for biliary leak: Fever, jaundice, shoulder pain, sepsis.
8. Monitor for biliary stricture: Jaundice, itching, abnormal bilirubin/ alkaline phosphatase.

Fast Facts

- Signs and symptoms specific to a liver transplant rejection are elevated liver function tests and hyperbilirubinemia.
- "Primary nonfunction" is the term used for liver graft failure occurring immediately post-op. The patient can become comatose and exhibit extreme coagulopathy, severely reduced urine output, jaundice, and/or very low glucose. Another transplant is the only way to reverse the condition.
- Complications specific to liver transplants include aphasia, acute liver failure, encephalopathy, myelinlysis biliary complications, and neuropathy.

HEART TRANSPLANT

Heart transplants may involve removal of the patient's damaged heart and replacing with the donated heart or leaving the patient's heart and "piggy-backing" the donor heart by connecting the chambers and blood vessels. In this manner, the donor heart assists the patient's damaged heart. Reasons for heart transplant include:

- Cardiomyopathy
- Coronary artery disease
- Congenital heart disease

Heart Transplant Guidelines

- Postoperative care is similar for any cardiac surgery patient, with some major differences.
  - Change in cardiac rhythm due to denervation of the donor heart
  - Potential for right ventricular failure
  - Administer prostaglandins, as ordered, to lower pulmonary vascular resistance
- Denervation of the donor heart
  - Loss of autonomic nervous system influence on the heart
  - Loss of vagal influence on the heart
  - Resting sinus rate is usually between 90 and 110 beats/min
  - Normal heart rate variations due to respiration do not occur

- Atropine is not effective on the transplanted heart
  - Dobutamine, epinephrine, and epicardial pacing may be required in the immediate postoperative period
- Increased heart rate, contractility, and cardiac output occur through circulating catecholamines
- Monitor for signs and symptoms of rejection

Fast Facts

Rejection of the heart is usually asymptomatic. Subtle signs may include decreased cardiac output, atrial dysrhythmias, low-grade fever, and elevated white blood cell count. Endomyocardial biopsy is performed weekly during the first postoperative month to monitor for rejection.

RECOVERY GUIDELINES FOR ORGAN TRANSPLANT RECIPIENTS

The vast majority of organ transplant patients are cared for in specialized transplant critical care units. Frequently, the patient arrives in the critical care unit directly from the operating room. Immunosuppresive medications are started immediately to prevent rejection. Generally, immunosuppression induction is started just prior to surgery.

The following assessments and interventions apply to most organ transplant recipients cared for in the critical care unit:

Assessment

- Complete head-to-toe assessment upon arrival to unit.
- Frequent physical and neurological reassessment.
- Ongoing assessment of fluid status; calculate fluid balance every 12 hours.
- Record input and output hourly and output each shift.
- Warm the patient to approximately 37°C.
- Manage pain adequately.
- Record daily weight.
- Assess for signs and symptoms of acute rejection such as fever, headache, nausea, vomiting, chills, malaise, and increased weight.
- With suspicion of rejection, anticipate an organ biopsy.
- Monitor lab values. Notify MD of abnormal results.

Respiratory

- Continuous monitoring of respiratory status, SaO_2, SpO_2, and arterial blood gases.
- Document the amount and appearance of chest tube drainage.
- Wean from the ventilator per MD orders. The extubation goal, for most transplant patients, is within 24 hours post-op.
- Use chest physiotherapy, incentive spirometry, and postural drainage; encourage coughing and deep breathing after extubation.
- Ensure completion of a daily chest x-ray.
- Elevate the head of the bed by 30°, unless contraindicated.
- Notify MD of chest tube drainage >200 mL in 1 hour.

Hemodynamic Monitoring

- Continuous monitoring of the EKG for changes; arrhythmias and dysrhythmias are common.
- Frequent monitoring of hemodynamics.
- Titrate vasoactive drips to maintain hemodynamics within ordered parameters.
- Administer diuretics, as ordered, to prevent fluid overload.

Infection Prevention

- Reverse isolation precautions, per the institution's policy.
- Maintain aseptic technique during IV and central line site care and dressing changes.
- Assess for signs/symptoms of infection.
- Infuse leukocyte depleted, cytomegalovirus-negative blood and blood products, as ordered, per the institution's protocol.
- Administer antibiotics, antifungals, and antivirals, as ordered.
- Administer immunosuppressive medications, as ordered. Examples include:
  - Alemtuzumab (Campath)
  - Azathioprine (Imuran)
  - Corticosteroids
  - Cychlophosphamide (Cytoxan)
  - Cyclosporine (Gengraf)
  - Mycophenolate mofetil (MMF)
  - Sirolimus (Rapamune)
  - Tacrolimus (FK-506)
- Review serum immunosuppressive drug levels. Determine whether they are within therapeutic range and notify MD.

Gastrointestinal

- Administer H2 blockers or proton pump inhibitors, as ordered.
- Evaluate GI status for possible paralytic ileus.
- Expect initiation of enteral feedings once bowel sounds return.

Routine Care

- Educate the patient regarding splinting of incision
- Turn the patient every 2 hours, unless contraindicated.
- Provide, or assist with, proper oral care.
- Perform range of motion exercises, as tolerated.
- Encourage mobilization and ambulation early, as tolerated.

Consultations

- Nutritionist
- Physical therapist
- Occupational therapist
- Wound care specialist
- Other members of the healthcare team as indicated
- Every transplant recipient requires post-op education, emotional support, and medical follow-up

Fast Facts

Immunosuppressive therapy has the potential to produce toxic side effects in almost every system of the body. Examples of how such toxicity might present include elevated blood glucose, coma, confusion, cortical blindness, encephalopathy, gingival hyperplasia, hyperkalemia, hypertension, leukopenia, quadriplegia, seizures, and tremors. Complications related to organ transplants include atelectasis, hemorrhage, infection, organ(s) rejection, paralytic ileus, pneumonia, renal failure, bleeding, and thrombosis.

REJECTION

Organ rejection can occur following any type of transplant. There are four major categories of organ rejection: hyperacute, accelerated, acute T-cell mediated, and chronic. Each category is treated differently, according to the underlying cause and symptoms.

The general symptoms associated with rejection are chills, diaphoresis, fever, exhaustion, hypertension, increased weight gain, poor appetite, tenderness at the graft site, peripheral edema, and a drop in urine output. Lab and diagnostic test results vary with the organ transplanted.

Hyperacute rejection happens almost immediately following the transplant and is often untreatable. Accelerated rejection happens within 2 to 5 days following the transplant and is managed with plasmapheresis and immunoglobulin G administration. Steroid and/or increased immunosuppression therapy is used to treat acute T-cell medicated rejection, which takes place within a few days to a few weeks following the transplant. Rejection that occurs months to a year after the transplant is generally chronic and not reversible. A gradual loss in organ/graft function is seen.

BECOMING A DONOR

Organ donation and transplantation saves lives. According to the U.S. Department of Health and Human Services, someone is added to the transplant waiting list every 10 minutes. On average, 95 transplant surgeries occur every day in the United States. One donor may be able to save eight lives. Consider becoming an organ donor. You can learn more and sign up at organdonor.gov.

Resources

Burns, S. M., & Delgado, S. A. (2019). *AACN essentials of critical care nursing* (4th ed.). New York, NY: McGraw-Hill.

Diepenbrock, N. H. (2015). *Quick reference to critical care* (5th ed.). Philadelphia, PA: Wolters Kluwer.

Health Resources & Services Administration. (n.d.). *This is national minority donor awareness week*. Retrieved from https://www.organdonor.gov/index.html

Hinkle, J. L., & Cheever, K. H. (2017). *Brunner & Suddarth's handbook of laboratory and diagnostic tests* (3rd ed.). Philadelphia, PA: Wolters Kluwer.

Jones, J., & Fix, B. (2015). *Critical care notes: Clinical pocket guide* (2nd ed.). Philadelphia, PA: F.A. Davis.

Morton, P. G., & Fontaine, D. K. (2018). *Critical care nursing: A holistic approach* (11th ed.). Philadelphia, PA: Wolters Kluwer.

Organ Procurement and Transplantation Network. (n.d.). *National data*. Retrieved from https://optn.transplant.hrsa.gov/data/view-data-reports/national-data/

United Network for Organ Sharing. (n.d.). Retrieved from https://unos.org/data/transplant-trends/

Urden, L. D., Stacy, K. M., & Lough, M. E. (2020). *Priorities in critical care nursing* (8th ed.). St. Louis, MO: Elsevier.

14

Burn and Integument Critical Care

According to the American Burn Association, approximately 486,000 patients were treated in the ED with burn-related injuries between 2011 and 2015. In 2016, 3,390 deaths occurred from burns sustained in a fire, with 2,800 of these from residential fires. Burn injuries may be caused by fire/flame, scalds, hot objects, electricity, and chemical means. These statistics and the fact that the integumentary system is the largest organ of the human body make education and skills regarding burn care an essential part of every ICU.

In this chapter, you will learn:

1. The types of burns
2. A description of the rule of nines
3. The classification guidelines for burns and corresponding nursing implementations
4. The signs and symptoms of smoke inhalation and carbon monoxide poisoning

BASIC BURN BREAKDOWN

A burn is simply a breakdown of the skin. The major types of burns include chemical, electrical, radiation, scald, and thermal burns. The severity of a burn is based on the percentage of body surface area (BSA) affected, the depth of the wound, the patient's age, the area of the body burned, the patient's medical history, accompanying injuries/issues, and the existence of an inhalation injury. Severity also increases with wounds to the eyes, ears, face, hands, feet, and groin.

THE RULE OF NINES

The determination of BSA involved in a burn is often done by the rule of nines, in which the body is broken down into percentage areas that are assessed for wounds. Once the assessment is complete, the total BSA affected can be calculated.

Fast Facts

Accepted percentages according to the rule of nines:

- Face and back of the head: 4.5% each
- Groin: 1%
- Lower back (buttocks): 9%
- Palms: 1% each
- Chest and back: 9% each
- Front or back of each arm: 4.5% each
- Abdomen: 9%
- Front or back of each leg: 9% each

Source: Data from Diepenbrock, N. H. (2015). *Quick reference to critical care* (5th ed.). Philadelphia, PA: Wolters Kluwer

An example of a burn BSA calculation by the rule of nines is a case in which the front of one leg (9%), the groin (1%), and the abdomen (9%) are burned. In this case, the total BSA involved is 19%.

BURN CLASSIFICATION

Burns are characterized by wound depth. Further classification includes the causative agent and the time and circumstances surrounding the burn.

- *Superficial:* Painful with pink/red skin, no blistering, possible minimal edema, and blanching. The epidermis is affected. Heals in 3 to 5 days with no scar.
- *Partial thickness:* Painful, with ink/red skin, blisters, weepy skin, and blanching. Epidermis and superficial dermis are affected. Heals in 2 to 3 weeks with possible scarring.

- *Deep partial thickness:* Painful, with pink/white dry skin, possible blisters, and no blanching. Epidermis, superficial dermis, and deep dermis are affected. Heals in 3 to 6 weeks with possible scarring.
- *Full thickness:* Actual wound is pain-free but surrounding area aches. Red/white/brown/black dry, leathery skin, and no blistering. All layers of the skin and subcutaneous tissue are affected; may include muscle, tendon, and/or bone. Eschar needs to be removed. Heals in >1 month and typically requires grafting. Scarring occurs.

TYPES OF BURNS

Chemical burns can cause tissue oxidation and denaturation, cellular dehydration and coagulation, and/or blistering. The symptoms are burning, pain, swelling, fluid loss, and/or discoloration. The severity and type of injury varies with the type of chemical exposure.

Electrical burns present with various symptoms. There may be white and/or leathery charring at the entrance and exit sites of the wound, the smell of burned skin, minimal or no pain, visual changes, seizures, and/or paralysis. EKG changes, such as ventricular fibrillation, asystole, nonspecific ST-segment changes, and sinus tachycardia, are often observed. Spinal cord trauma is possible. Rhabdomyolosis may be present. The iceberg effect—small wound sites with a large amount of internal damage—is often noted.

Radiation burns are not common. These injuries affect the DNA and have a long-term impact. The immediate injury site exhibits characteristics similar to a wound.

Scalds occur from contact with hot steam or liquid. Children are most commonly treated for this type of burn. The appearance of such wounds ties in closely with the classification descriptions.

Thermal burns are caused by flames or contact with something extremely hot. These wounds fit the classification descriptions very closely.

INHALATION ISSUES

An inhalation injury from steam, smoke, or chemicals is frequently characterized by shortness of breath, hoarseness, chest tightness, rapid respirations, singed nares, gray or black sputum, facial burns, and/or stridor.

Carbon monoxide poisoning is characterized by hallmark cherry-red skin. Symptoms also include confusion, nausea, syncope, headache, changes in vision, and an increased carboxyhemoglobin

(COHb) level (generally >10%). Carbon monoxide poisoning is often experienced when smoke exposure occurs in a small, confined area. Severe cases may be treated with hyperbaric oxygen.

Fast Facts

Burn victims cared for in the ICU usually meet the following criteria:

- Over 20% total BSA affected
- Full thickness burns
- Comorbidities, such as cardiovascular disease, diabetes, or kidney disease
- Inhalation or high-voltage electrical injury
- Additional injuries requiring ICU intervention

STAGES OF BURN CARE

Care of the patient with burns is classified into two stages: the resuscitative and acute phases. Management depends on the location and extent of the burn injury. The resuscitative phase begins at the time of the injury and in the emergency department. It generally lasts between 48 and 72 hours. The acute phase is characterized by:

- Loss of capillary integrity with increased permeability of the capillary membrane
- Fluid shift to the interstitial spaces
- Decreased cardiac output, blood pressure, renal blood flow, and urine output
- Increased heart rate and peripheral vasoconstriction
- Hyperkalemia
- Red blood cell lysis with hematuria, anemia, and myoglobinuria (may result in rhabdomyolysis)
- Increased clotting time and prothrombin time
- Metabolic acidosis
- Hypothermia

After the patient is stabilized and out of the acute phase, the resuscitative phase begins. This phase is characterized by the onset of diuresis and:

- Capillary membrane stability with return of fluids to the intravascular space
- Hemodilution with reduced electrolyte and hematocrit levels (dilutional)

Fast Facts

Carefully monitor potassium levels as the patient moves out of the acute phase and into the resuscitative phase. Hypokalemia is a risk as potassium moves back into the cell.

BURN TREATMENT

Complications associated with burns can be severe, including shock, kidney failure, respiratory distress/failure, sepsis, and limb loss. Burn management focuses on preventing complications.

The major goal during the initial treatment of a burn patient is fluid resuscitation. There are two methods to calculate the amount of fluid to be infused:

1. Parkland formula: Lactated Ringers – 4 mL × body weight in kg × %BSA burned. Infuse half of this amount over the first 8 hours and the remainder over the next 16 hours.
2. Modified Brooke formula: 2 mL × body weight in kg × %BSA burned. Infuse half of this amount over the first 8 hours and the remainder over the next 16 hours.

There is a marked difference in the amount of fluid in these two formulae. As a rule, the amount should be guided by the type and degree of burn, as well as other conditions such as an intoxicated patient and comorbidities. Monitoring urine output with an output of 0.5 to 1 mL/kg/h is a common resuscitation goal. During the second 24 hours postinjury, colloids may be infused at 0.5 mL of colloid × weight in kg × % BSA burned. Refer to your institution's protocol.

The following are the guidelines and implementations for ICU burn treatment.

Respiratory and Airway Management

- Maintain a patent airway and prepare for intubation.
- Maintain SpO_2 >95%.
- Monitor arterial blood gases.
- Assess sputum for color, thickness, and odor.
- Administer bronchodilators, as ordered.
- Perform chest physiotherapy, as ordered.
- Ensure chest x-ray completion.
- Turn, cough, and deep breathing; and incentive spirometry when extubated.

Fast Facts

Carefully monitor airway patency of nonintubated patients. Laryngeal edema may develop up to 72 hours postinjury.

For patients with increased COHb, provide 100% FiO_2, as ordered

Assessment and Hemodynamic Stability

- Perform a complete head-to-toe assessment upon arrival to the unit.
- Maintain mean arterial pressure >60 mmHg via fluid infusion or vasoactive medication administration, as ordered.
- Anticipate the insertion of a ventral venous line and/or pulmonary artery catheter.
- Administer blood/blood products, as ordered, according to the institution's protocol.
- Closely monitor fluid status, and measure input and output every hour. Urine output should be 30 to 50 mL/h. Urine output for electrical burn victims should be >100 mL/h.
- Insert nasogastric tube, as ordered.
- Test gastric pH. Assess for blood in emesis, nasogastric drainage, and/or stool.
- Initiate stress ulcer and deep vein thrombosis prophylaxis per protocol.
- Observe for the signs/symptoms of abdominal compartment syndrome such as poor ventilation and reduced urine output during fluid administration.
- Document daily weight.
- Assess complete blood count, electrolytes, albumin, blood glucose, BUN, creatinine, osmolality, prothrombin time/international normalized ratio, partial thromboplastin time, and urine-specific gravity.
- Review medical history for tetanus administration. If none is found, administer tetanus shot, as ordered.
- Maintain room temperature between 85 and 90°F.
- Maintain the head of the bed at least 30° to 45°. Elevate burned extremities.

Perform/assist with range of motion exercises to prevent contractures. Care of the burn patient requires a multidisciplinary team approach. The team should include a dietitian, physical therapist, occupational therapist, psychiatrist/mental health worker, social services, wound care specialist, and pharmacist. Patients experiencing

BOX 14.1 BURN/WOUND CARE GUIDELINES

- For a chemical burn, ensure complete removal of the chemical from the body. Do not rub skin; blot or brush should also be avoided
- Premedicate with analgesics prior to wound care. Alert and oriented patients may use a patient-controlled analgesia pump.
- Perform wound care daily or twice a day, as ordered:
  - Cleanse and debride, as ordered, using aseptic technique.
  - Clip hair around the site.
  - Provide wound care, as ordered. Wounds may be left open or closed (covered with a topical medication and dressed).
- Assess burn site for drainage, and document appearance, color, and odor.
- Assess wound for changes in appearance, margins, or drainage.
- Perform wound culture, as ordered.
- Cover partial thickness wounds to reduce pain.
- Topical medications that may be ordered include:
  - Silver sulfadiazine 1% (Silvadene)
  - Mafenide acetate 5% or 10% (Sulfamylon)
  - Silver nitrate 0.5%
  - Silver sheeting (Acticoat)
  - Mupirocin (Bactroban)

extensive burns may require frequent wound excision and/or skin grafts. For full thickness and/or circumferential burns, an escharotomy or fasciotomy may be indicated. Depending on the extent of the burn, artificial skin products may be required. Burn patients require enhanced nutritional intake to support increased energy needs for wound healing (see Box 14.1).

Fast Facts

Burn patients are at an increased risk of infection. Infection prevention guidelines for burn patients include maintaining contact isolation precautions, as well as providing dedicated equipment for each patient, including stethoscope, thermometers, and blood pressure cuffs.

Resources

Burns, S. M., & Delgado, S. A. (2019). *AACN essentials of critical care nursing* (4th ed.). New York, NY: McGraw-Hill.

Hinkle, J. L., & Cheever, K. H. (2017). *Brunner & Suddarth's handbook of laboratory and diagnostic tests* (3rd ed.). Philadelphia, PA: Wolters Kluwer.

Jones, J., & Fix, B. (2015). *Critical care notes: Clinical pocket guide* (2nd ed.). Philadelphia, PA: F.A. Davis.

Morton, P. G., & Fontaine, D. K. (2018). *Critical care nursing: A holistic approach* (11th ed.). Philadelphia, PA: Wolters Kluwer.

Urden, L. D., Stacy, K. M., & Lough, M. E. (2020). *Priorities in critical care nursing* (8th ed.). St. Louis, MO: Elsevier.

Reference

Diepenbrock, N. H. (2015). *Quick reference to critical care* (5th ed.). Philadelphia, PA: Wolters Kluwer.

III

Patient- and Family-Centered Care

15

Withdrawal of Treatment and Terminal Extubation

Emotional support is a key component of end-of-life (EOL) care and is important for the patient, family, caregivers, and ICU staff. Certain strategies and guidelines can help ease the stress and emotional turmoil associated with imminent death and EOL care. Guidelines for the withdrawal of treatment, palliative care, and the generalized protocol for a terminal wean can help facilitate a "good" death.

In this chapter, you will learn:

1. The guidelines for the withdrawal of medical treatment
2. The general protocol for a "terminal wean"
3. How to emotionally support patients and family when death is imminent
4. Self-care guidelines for nurses providing EOL care

WITHDRAWAL OF MEDICAL TREATMENT

Over the last several years, there has been an increasing focus on care for dying patients and their families. Critical care nurses and physicians focus on life-saving, sometimes using heroic measures. Improved technology and medications have the ability to prolong life. However, death is inevitable, and there is now increased attention on the human experience of dying. In 2014, the Institute of

Medicine (IOM) released "Dying in America: Improving Quality and Honoring Individual Preferences Near the End of Life." This landmark study identified five recommendations to improve EOL care:

1. Delivery of person-centered, family-oriented EOL care
2. Clinician–patient communication and advance care planning
3. Professional education and development
4. Policies and payment systems to support high-quality EOL care
5. Public education and engagement

Once the physicians and the patient's family and/or healthcare proxy decide that additional medical interventions will be futile, medical treatment can be withdrawn. This includes ventilation support, nutrition, IV fluids, antibiotics, and/or blood products. Withdrawal of medical treatment is emotional for both the family and the staff.

Prior to withdrawal of treatment, the physicians, nurses, clergy, social workers, and other hospital support staff should provide clear details to family members regarding the process and allow them time to absorb this information. Some clinicians suggest using the term *choosing comfort* or *care and comfort* because families tend to find it easier to understand these terms as they are less emotionally taxing than some others.

Fast Facts

To help the family cope with the situation, assure them that:

1. The cause of death is the underlying disease and not the withdrawal of treatment.
2. Medication will be administered to maintain the patient's comfort and prevent suffering.
3. Staff will continue to care for the patient. The patient will not be neglected.

TERMINAL WEAN

The withdrawal of ventilator support from an incurably ill patient is often referred to as a terminal wean. For the family, the nurse usually follows these guidelines:

■ Rely on a properly trained nurse and respiratory therapist who perform this procedure at the patient's bedside.

- Determine whether family members wish to remain with the patient during the terminal wean and extubation process and spend time with the patient after death. These questions should be asked in a caring, understanding, and nonjudgmental manner.
- Ensure that the room is as comfortable as possible. Provide chairs, tissues, and as much privacy as possible. Be readily available to address the family's needs and/or provide comfort measures and medications for the patient.
- Facilitate any family requests for spiritual/clergy support.
- Prepare the family for what to expect during the terminal wean process in a clear, concise, caring manner.
- If the patient is dependent on the ventilator and vasopressors, death typically follows as soon as the support is removed.
- Encourage family members to touch and speak to the patient and express any feelings they are experiencing. After the patient expires, allow the family to spend time in the room.

The facility and its practitioners follow a specific protocol, which usually includes:

- Document conversations with the family and other healthcare team members.
- Consider organ donation prior to treatment withdrawal.
- Maintain IV access site for palliative care medication administration.
- Remove monitoring equipment not needed for patient comfort.
- Disable or mute alarms on the monitor and ventilator.
- Hold all neuromuscular blocking medications, providing adequate reversal time.
- Administer pain/anxiety medications 30 minutes prior to the initiation of ventilator withdrawal.
- Remove restraints.
- Decide between gradual or immediate ventilator withdrawal:
  - Gradual ventilator withdrawal: Reduction of the respiratory rate (RR) of the ventilator by 2 to 3 breaths per minute, at 15-minute intervals, until the RR of the ventilator is zero. Next, reduce positive end expiratory pressure (PEEP) and pressure support (PS) until the patient exhibits spontaneous respiration.
  - Immediate ventilator withdrawal: The ventilator is withdrawn without changes in RR, PEEP, or PS.
- Position patient upright, whenever possible.
- Administer antisecretory medication such as hycoscyamine (Anaspaz), if ordered.
- Administer haloperidol (Haldol) or midazolam (Versed) for terminal restlessness, if ordered.

- Begin weaning ventilator settings.
- Continuously monitor the patient for signs and symptoms of pain, respiratory distress, agitation, or anxiety.
- Administer medications for pain, respiratory distress, agitation, and/or anxiety, as needed, to keep the patient comfortable.
- Extubate the patient, if ordered.
- Deactivate pacemakers and implanted cardioverter-defibrillators.
- Notify the physician when spontaneous respirations have ceased.

Fast Facts

Withdrawal of ventilator support for a patient is rarely a medical examiner's case. If it is, follow hospital protocol for removal of lines, chest, and endotracheal tubes, and any other applicable modality before, during, and after withdrawal of medical treatment.

Resources

Burns, S. M., & Delgado, S. A. (2019). *AACN essentials of critical care nursing* (4th ed.). New York, NY: McGraw-Hill.

Campbell, M. L. (2018). Ensuring breathing comfort at the end of life: The integral role of the critical care nurse. *American Journal of Critical Care, 27*(4), 264–269. doi:10.4037/ajcc2018420. Retrieved from https://www.aacn.org/docs/cemedia/a1827043.pdf

The Institute of Medicine. (2014). *Annual report.*

Morton, P. G., & Fontaine, D. K. (2018). *Critical care nursing: A holistic approach* (11th ed.). Philadelphia, PA: Wolters Kluwer.

Pizzo, P. A., & Walker, D. M. (2014). *Dying in America: Improving quality and honoring individual preferences near the end of life.* Washington, DC: Institute of Medicine.

Urden, L. D., Stacy, K. M., & Lough, M. E. (2020). *Priorities in critical care nursing* (8th ed.). St. Louis, MO: Elsevier.

16

Palliative Care in the ICU

Although palliative care principles should be initiated at the time of the diagnosis, the integration of these principles in the critical care unit may improve the quality of death and dying for patients at the end of life. Critical care nurses provide coordinated services and communication to the patient and family during very difficult times.

In this chapter, you will learn:

1. The difference between palliative care and hospice care
2. Implementation of a palliative care bundle
3. Definition of End of Life Nursing Education Consortium (ELNEC)
4. Emotional care for the critical care nurse

PALLIATIVE CARE

Palliative care is an interdisciplinary holistic approach to care for patients with serious illnesses such as:

- Heart failure
- Chronic obstructive pulmonary disease
- Cancer
- Dementia
- Parkinson's disease

Initiate palliative care at the time of the diagnosis, even when conventional medical treatment and therapies are in place. Over time, and

Table 16.1

Differences Between Palliative Care and Hospice Care

	Palliative Care	Hospice Care
Who can be treated?	Anyone with a serious illness	Anyone with a serious illness with 6 months or less to live
Symptom relief	Yes	Yes
Curative treatments	Yes	No. Care is focused on symptom relief

Source: Adapted from Anderson, W. G., & Puntillo, K. (2017). Palliative care professional development for critical care nurses: A multicenter program. *American Journal of Critical Care, 26*(5), 361–371. doi:10.4037/ajcc2017336 and National Institute on Aging. (n.d.). *What are palliative care and hospice care?* Retrieved from https://www.nia.nih.gov/health/what-are-palliative-care-and-hospice-care#palliative

as the disease progresses, palliative care may transition into hospice care. Implementing palliative care principles at the early stages of a disease provides the patient time to express desires and communicate care preferences and plan.

Palliative care is distinctively different from hospice care. In palliative care, treatment continues for the underlying disease. In hospice care, treatment of the disease is discontinued and the focus is on symptom relief. Hospice care is generally initiated when the patient has approximately 6 months or less to live. See Table 16.1 for the differences between palliative care and hospice care.

Palliative care is the active total care of patients with an advanced illness. During this phase of critical care, the focus shifts to the patient's quality of life and comfort level. A multidisciplinary palliative care team works to make the patient and the family as comfortable as possible.

Members of the palliative care team may include:

- Registered nurse
- Case manager
- Social worker
- Hospital chaplain
- Pharmacist
- Dietitian
- Physician

Through evidence-based practice, a palliative care bundle has been developed for critical care. This bundle is an interdisciplinary approach focusing on specific activities of care on days 1, 3, and 5 of critical care admission.

Day 1:

- Identify the patient's decision-maker.
- Address any advance directives.
- Address the CPR or "code" status.
- Assess and manage pain symptoms.
- Conduct a palliative care screen.
- Arrange a family meeting.

Day 3:

- Social worker assessment.
- Spiritual care assessment.

Day 5:

- Conduct an interdisciplinary family meeting.

If the patient is able, discuss requests and preferences. Questions to be considered include:

- Is there an advance directive?
- Who is the patient's healthcare proxy or spokesperson?
- Are specific family members to visit?
- Does the patient want any religious and/or cultural practices to be observed?

Encourage the patient to express any emotions that they are experiencing. Listen in an open manner, and answer questions honestly.

ADVANCE DIRECTIVES

Advance directives are specific instructions directing healthcare when patients are no longer able to speak for themselves. Generally, it is a written document sometimes referred to as a living will or durable power of attorney for healthcare. Refer to your state-specific guidelines and laws surrounding advance directives. Everyone is encouraged to have an advance directive and to identify a specific person to speak on your behalf. The patient's advance directive should become part of the medical chart.

SYMPTOM MANAGEMENT IN PALLIATIVE CARE

In the critical care unit, managing the symptoms that patients encounter during end-of-life care is paramount. Pain, dyspnea, restlessness, and/or terminal delirium are the major symptoms that occur. Skin care is also a priority with these patients.

Pain is treated with a combination of medications. Nonsteroidal anti-inflammatory drugs (NSAIDs), opioids (primarily morphine), and corticosteroids are used to treat pain during palliative care. Antidepressants are also often administered to relieve neuropathic pain. Try to identify and eradicate the sources of pain. Undertreatment of pain is often reported by family members; however, this is not an acceptable outcome. Vigilance regarding pain control is required when providing palliative care.

Position the patient for comfort and reassess frequently for pain. Because the patient is often unable to express pain on a 1 to 10 scale, observe facial expressions, respirations, moaning or groaning, and consolability. During end-of-life (EOL) care, dosages of certain medications, such as morphine, may exceed those in general critical care nursing practice.

Dyspnea occurs in almost all patients undergoing EOL care. This is uncomfortable for the patient to experience and for the family to observe. Diuretics and morphine reduce congestion, while anxiolytics help reduce anxiety. A trial of low-dose oxygen may reduce dyspnea; however, it is not used to improve oxygen saturation levels. Position the patient upright on the bed, if possible, to maximize lung capacity. One inch of nitroglycerin paste applied to the chest wall may improve orthopnea. Hycoscyamine sulfate can be given to help reduce audible secretions. If wheezing is noted, bronchodilators are often administered.

Proper skin care and hygiene are essential during EOL care as they maximize comfort and assure both the patient and the family that care is ongoing. Follow ICU skin care protocols. Bathe the patient daily and apply skin protectants and/or moisturizers, as needed. Turn the patient every 2 hours or as needed, based on pain and/or discomfort. Use a low-pressure mattress system, if available and if the patient condition dictates need. Provide frequent oral care.

Patients undergoing EOL care often exhibit terminal delirium and restlessness. Other signs and symptoms include nonpurposeful motor activity, changing level of consciousness, cognitive failure, agitation, and hallucinations. Haloperidol (Haldol), olanzapine (Zyprexa), risperidone (Risperdal), midazolam (Versed), and/or chlorpromazine (Thorazine) may be administered, if ordered, to combat these symptoms and provide comfort to the patient.

Fast Facts

A patient close to death may experience nearing-death awareness (NDA). Deceased loved ones may appear to the patient and "speak." Other visions might also occur. NDA is different from terminal

(continued)

(continued)

delirium, primarily because the patient is not distressed or afraid of the visions. Their message is usually symbolic and might also be directed to family members. Explain to them and the patient that this type of experience is normal.

EMOTIONAL SUPPORT OF THE FAMILY

Frequently, once care turns to palliation in the ICU, the patient's health status has progressed to such a serious point that the patient is no longer able to make decisions. The family then becomes the focus of the healthcare team's emotional support. Provide education regarding care, symptoms, and medical management to the family. Assure them that medications will be provided to alleviate pain and anxiety and that the patient will not be neglected because of the choice to withhold or withdraw medical treatment. A comfortable environment encourages family members to interact with and care for the patient. Allow them to express all emotions.

EOL care involves many clinical skills and requires positive emotional support for the patient and family. Remember to:

1. Allow family members to spend as much time as possible with the patient prior to and after death.
2. Provide family access to clergy or other spiritual advisors if they request it. Attempt to honor the religious practices of the patient and family.
3. Be emotionally and physically available to discuss the patient's status, providing full disclosure of the situation.
4. Provide time for family members to ask questions, express emotions, and grieve.
5. Invite the family to participate in the final care following death of their loved one. Some family members will appreciate this opportunity.
6. Be sensitive to the possibility that a family member might need to actually hear medical personnel state that the patient has expired.
7. Offer follow-up care that might include:
   a. A meeting of the family and physician or healthcare team.
   b. A simple card or phone call from the healthcare team.
   c. Information about the facility's bereavement program and support groups for those who have experienced the death of a loved one.
   d. Contact with a social worker for referral to posthospital emotional support.

HEALTHCARE TEAM EMOTIONAL SUPPORT

Working in the critical care unit is physically demanding and emotionally taxing. It is a labor of love. Nurses, as well as the rest of the healthcare team, are concerned about the patients and families they care for and tend to forget about their own needs, especially when dealing with EOL issues such as organ donation, withdrawal of medical treatment, and palliative care.

Critical care nurses must remember to take steps necessary to support their own physical and emotional health. Education regarding end-of-life care protocols and expectations is one way to improve the understanding of the dying process. Actually participating in such care produces positive experiences related to patient and family comfort and satisfaction. Some important considerations include:

1. Exercising moderately, eating a well-balanced diet, and staying hydrated to maintain physical health and support the ability to provide excellent care
2. Participating in activities outside of work, enjoying hobbies, and relaxing with friends and family to maintain positive emotional health
3. The support of clergy, social workers, bereavement counselors, and psychosocial support staff to improve coping skills, find emotional release, and manage grief

ELNEC provides education for nurses providing palliative and EOL care. It consists of the following six modules:

1. Nursing Care at the End of Life
2. Pain Management
3. Symptom Management
4. Communication
5. Loss, Grief, Bereavement
6. Preparation for and Care at the Time of Death

ELNEC-Critical Care is specifically designed for critical care practitioners and the unique challenges of providing or initiating palliative care in the critical care unit. All critical care nurses are strongly encouraged to take advantage of this continuing education.

Resources

American Association of Colleges of Nursing. (n.d.). Retrieved from https://www.aacnnursing.org/Portals/42/ELNEC/PDF/FactSheet.pdf

Morton, P. G., & Fontaine, D. K. (2018). *Critical care nursing: A holistic approach* (11th ed.). Philadelphia, PA: Wolters Kluwer.

Toumbs, R., Cossey, T., Taylor, T., & Choi, H. (2019). Standardizing communications improves use of palliative care in patients with stroke. *The Journal for Nurse Practitioners, 15*(5), e89–e92. doi:10.1016/j.nurpra.2018.12.019

References

Anderson, W. G., & Puntillo, K. (2017). Palliative care professional development for critical care nurses: A multicenter program. *American Journal of Critical Care, 26*(5), 361–371. doi:10.4037/ajcc2017336

National Institute on Aging. (n.d.). *What are palliative care and hospice care?* Retrieved from https://www.nia.nih.gov/health/what-are-palliative-care-and-hospice-care#palliative

17

Organ Donation

*According to federal legislation, hospitals must identify poten-
tial organ donors. Additionally, The Joint Commission has a
standard addressing organ donation. Although an imminent
death is a very difficult time for the family, the request for organ
donation may be made by an organ procurement specialist who
has training on making supportive requests. Even though solid
organ donation may not be possible, eye or tissue donation may
be an option.*

In this chapter, you will learn:

1. The number of individuals awaiting organ transplant
2. General organ donation and procurement guidelines
3. Meaning of the "Honor Walk" for organ donor patients

EYE AND ORGAN DONATION

According to the United Network for Organ Sharing (UNOS), there
are over 110,000 people in the United States awaiting an organ
transplant. The waiting list grows longer each day, while the number of potential donors does not. The reasons for the low number of
donors are numerous, and many myths and misconceptions abound.
Examples of myths and misconceptions, which medical professionals
know are unfounded, include the following:

1. If a physician knows that a patient is an organ donor, he or she
   will not work as hard to save the patient.

2. Being rich and famous improves a patient's place on the transplant list.
3. Listing "organ donor" on a driver's license or having a donor card is all that is needed to be a donor.
4. The only organs that can be transplanted are the heart, liver, and/or kidneys.
5. Most patients with a medical history are not fit to donate organs.
6. Older patients are not eligible to donate organs.
7. The family of the donor is charged a fee if organs are donated.
8. If the organs of a patient are donated, the body is changed in such a way that it is unsuitable for viewing at the funeral.
9. Most religions do not allow organ donation.

Fast Facts

While a patient may not be suitable for heart donation, other organs can often be used, such as the corneas, lungs, liver, pancreas, kidneys, skin, bone, bone marrow, cartilage, tendons, fascia, and/or dura mater.

It is the responsibility of the hospital staff, local and state organ bank representatives, and UNOS to educate patients, family members, and the public. According to federal law, Medicare, and The Joint Commission, there are specific requirements hospitals must follow:

1. Hospitals have written protocols guiding organ and tissue donation.
2. Surviving family members have the opportunity to designate organ and tissue donation.

Critical care nurses often encounter situations where eye and/or organ donation is a possibility. Provide emotional support and education to the family while attempting to honor the patient's wishes, either for or against donation. According to the 2006 Universal Anatomical Gift Act (UAGA), organs of a patient who indicated prior to death that he or she wished to participate in organ donation, such as on a driver's license, must be considered for donation. The UAGA also specifies that if a patient previously signed a refusal for eye and/or organ donation, family members or the healthcare proxy cannot override the patient's wishes and should not be requested to do so.

Once it is clear that a patient requested to be a donor or if there is no indication of the patient's wishes in this regard, medical suitability for eye and/or organ donation must be considered before approaching the family to prevent undue emotional distress.

Fast Facts

Some people request that their body be donated to "science" for medical research. Most research centers accept bodies and organs regardless of the illness, pathology, or cause of death. A person usually has contact information for the facility that will be accepting his or her body detailed in an advance directive.

ORGAN DONATION AND PROCUREMENT GUIDELINES

Most hospitals have policies outlining their organ donation/procurement process. Some general guidelines are as follows:

1. A potential organ donor is identified.
2. An organ procurement organization (OPO), such as a state organ center or eye bank, is notified that a death is imminent. Discuss the patient's status with family members in an open, unbiased manner to allow them time to make informed decisions regarding eye and organ donation, as well as to express emotions about the patient's imminent death. Answer all questions honestly. Seek help from the OPO, if needed.
3. When the OPO is contacted, the medical team caring for the patient is asked various questions, including the patient's age, current status, and medical history, to determine preliminary suitability for donation.
4. A physician who meets the healthcare institution's guidelines for appropriate skill sets, training, and expertise regarding neurological status must declare brain death, which is defined as an irreversible loss of all brain function, based on both clinical and radiological evidence. A second opinion may be required.
5. Written consent is completed and witnessed once the family has had time to process the situation with support and education from the OPO representative, hospital staff, and/or clergy. A release from the medical examiner may also be required. Once this paperwork is complete, the patient is officially a "donor."

6. The donor's true medical suitability must be determined through a detailed medical and social history, a complete organ systems review, and lab work. OPOs and eye, organ, and tissue banks help this process proceed smoothly.

7. Donor management care must be provided throughout the evaluation period. Medications, respiratory care, and IV fluids are given to the donor to maximize the integrity of the organs and tissues for procurement.

8. The organ procurement procedure is performed using sterile technique once medical suitability is determined. The organs are preserved with a solution, and then transferred into sterile bags and stored on ice in coolers. Specially trained transplant teams are used to transport the organs according to OPO directions. Tissue recovery occurs in a similar manner after viable organs have been procured.

9. Disposition of the donor's body occurs according to institution's guidelines and the wishes of the patient and/or family.

10. Prompt follow-up occurs, with OPOs sending a letter to the donor's family detailing information about the recipients of their loved one's organs. Information regarding the organ recipients and the amazing outcome of the hard work completed by the team is provided to the facility and staff where the organs were harvested. The recipients' identities are not revealed.

Grief counseling is often available to donor families. Some OPOs have ceremonies throughout the year to honor the extraordinary gift of life that the donor and family provided.

Recently, many hospitals have started implementing the "Walk of Honor" or "Honor Walk," where hospital employees line the hallways as the patient is slowly transported to the operating room. This is a very solemn and respectful way to acknowledge the patient and the family.

Resources

Diepenbrock, N. H. (2015). *Quick reference to critical care* (5th ed.). Philadelphia, PA: Wolters Kluwer.

Jones, J., & Fix, B. (2015). *Critical care notes: Clinical pocket guide* (2nd ed.). Philadelphia, PA: F.A. Davis.

Morton, P. G., & Fontaine, D. K. (2018). *Critical care nursing: A holistic approach* (11th ed.). Philadelphia, PA: Wolters Kluwer.

Urden, L. D., Stacy, K. M., & Lough, M. E. (2016). *Priorities in critical care nursing* (7th ed.). St. Louis, MO: Elsevier.

Appendix A: Common Lab Values[*]

Arterial Blood Gas	
pH:	7.35–7.45
pO$_2$:	80–100 mmHg
pCO$_2$:	35–45 mmHg
HCO$_3$:	22–26 mEq/L
Base Excess:	–2 to +2
O$_2$ Sat:	>95%

Cardiac Markers			
CK-MB	Male: 0–4.2 ng/mL	Myocardial infarction:	Onset: 3–6 hours
	Female: 0–3.1 ng/mL		Peak: 12–24 hours
			Elevated: 2–3 days
Troponin		Myocardial infarction:	>2.0 ng/mL

[*]Always refer to your institution's lab ranges for normal values.

Comprehensive Metabolic Panel

Na	135–145 mEq/L	
K	3.5–5.3 mEq/L	
Cl	99–111 mEq/L	
CO_2	22–26 mEq/L	
BUN	10–23 mcg/dL	
Creatinine	0.6–1.3 mg/dL	
Glucose	70–115 mg/dL	
Calcium	8.5–10.2 mg/dL	
Phosphorus	2.5–4.9 mg/dL	
Magnesium	1.8–2.4 mg/dL	
ALT	Male: 19–36 units/L	Female: 24–36 units/L
Albumin	3.7–5.1 g/dL	
ALKP	Male: 35–142 units/L	Female: 25–125 units/L
AST	Male: 20–40 units/L	Female: 15–30 units/L
Bilirubin, total	0.1–1.2 mg/dL	
Protein, total	6–8 g/dL	

Complete Blood Count

RBC	Male: $4.7–6.1 \times 10^6/mm^3$	Female: $4.2–5.4 \times 10^6/mm^3$
Hgb	Male: 14–18 g/dL	Female: 12–16 g/dL
Hct	Male: 42–52%	Female: 37–47%
WBC	$4.8–10.8 \times 10^3/mm^3$	
Platelets	$150–450 \times 10^3/mm^3$	
Eosinophils	1%–7%	
Basophils	0%–1%	
Lymphocytes	24%–44%	
Monocytes	3%–10%	
Neutrophils	40%–80%	
Bands	0%–6%	

Urinalysis

Specific gravity	1.003–1.030
pH	4.5–7.5
Protein	Negative
Leukocytes	Negative
Glucose	Negative
Ketones	Negative
Nitrate	Negative
Bilirubin	Negative

Coagulation

Bleeding time	4–7 minutes
D-dimer	Negative
Fibrinogen	200–400 mg/dL
Fibrin split product	<10 mcg/dL
INR	2.0–3.0
PT	11–14 sec
PTT	<40 sec

ALKP, alkaline phosphatase; ALT, alanine aminotransferase; AST, aspartate aminotransferase; BUN, blood urea nitrogen; CK-MB, creatine kinase-muscle/brain; Hct, hematocrit; Hgb, hemoglobin; INR, international normalized ratio; PT, prothrombin time; PTT, partial thromboplastin time; RBC, red blood cell; WBC, white blood cell.

Resources

Bladh, V. L. (2019). *Davis's comprehensive manual of laboratory and diagnostic tests with nursing implications* (8th ed.). Philadelphia, PA: FA Davis.

Hinkle, J. L., & Cheever, K. H. (2017). *Brunner & Suddarth's Handbook of Laboratory and Diagnostic Tests* (3rd ed.). Philadelphia, PA: Wolters Kluwer.

Appendix B:
Hemodynamic Parameters

Parameter	Normal Range	Formula
CO	4–8 L/min	SV × HR
CI	2.5–4.3 L/min/m²	CO ÷ BSA
MAP	70–105 mmHg	2 (DBP) + SBP ÷ 3
RAP	2–8 mmHg	
PAOP	8–12 mmHg	
Pulmonary artery systolic	15–35 mmHg	
Pulmonary artery diastolic	10–15 mmHg	
Pulmonary vascular resistance	100–250 dynes/s/cm^{-5}	PAM − PAOP × 80 ÷ CO
Pulmonary vascular resistance index	255–285 dynes/s/cm^{-5}/m²	PAM − PAOP × 80 ÷ CI
PAM	15–20 mmHg	
Systemic vascular resistance	800–1200 dynes/s/cm^{-5}	MAP − RAP × 80 ÷ CO
Systemic vascular resistance index	1970–2390 dynes/s/cm^{-5}/m²	MAP − RAP × 80 ÷ CI

(continued)

Parameter	Normal Range	Formula
SV	50–100 mL/beat	CO/HR × 1,000
Ejection fraction	>60%	
Mixed venous saturation	60–80%	

BSA, body surface area; CI, cardiac index; CO, cardiac output; DBP: diastolic blood pressure; MAP, mean arterial pressure; PAM, pulmonary artery mean; PAOP, pulmonary artery wedge; RAP, right atrial pressure; SBP, systolic blood pressure; SV, stroke volume.

Resources

Burns, S. M., & Delgado, S. A. (2019). *AACN essentials of critical care nursing* (4th ed.). New York, NY: McGraw-Hill.

Diepenbrock, N. H. (2015). *Quick reference to critical care* (5th ed.). Philadelphia, PA: Wolters Kluwer.

Jones, J., & Fix, B. (2015). *Critical care notes: Clinical pocket guide* (2nd ed.). Philadelphia, PA: FA Davis.

Urden, L. D., Stacy, K. M., & Lough, M. E. (2020). *Priorities in critical care nursing* (8th ed.). St. Louis, MO: Elsevier.

Appendix C: Common Critical Care IV Medications

generic/Trade	Classification and Indication	Dosage
Vasopressors		
dobutamine/Dobutrex	Cardiac stimulant; beta-1 agonist Cardiac surgery and organic heart disease	2.5–10 mcg/kg/min to maximum dose 40 mcg/kg/min
dopamine/Intropin	Adrenergic Increase renal perfusion, shock, hypotension; dose-dependent response	2.5 mcg/kg/min to maximum dose 50 mcg/kg/min Low dose (renal): 1–3 mcg/kg/min Medium ($\uparrow$ contractility): 3–10 mcg/kg/min Medium (vasoconstriction): >10 mcg/kg/min High (similar to Levophed): >20 mcg/kg/min
fenoldopam/Corlopam	Vasodilator; anti-hypertensive Hypertensive crisis, malignant HTN	0.01–1.6 mcg/kg/min
milrinone/Primacor	Inotropic, vasodilator Short-term management of advanced heart failure not responding to other medications	Bolus: 50 mcg/kg over 10 min; follow with 0.375–0.75 mcg/kg/min

(continued)

generic/Trade	Classification and Indication	Dosage
nesiritide/Natrecor	Vasodilator Coronary vasodilation; chronic stable angina; heart failure associated with AMI	Bolus: 2 mcg/kg; follow with 0.01 mcg/kg/min
nitroglycerin	Vasodilator Antianginal	5 mcg/min, titrate by 5 mcg/min every 3–5 min to 20 mcg/min to chest pain relief; then increase by 10–20 mcg/min
nicardipine/Cardene	Antianginal; calcium channel blocker; acute HTN for short-term use only	Acute HTN: 5 mg/hr increasing by 2.5 mg/hr every 5–15 min, titrate for BP; max dose 15 mg/hr
nitroprusside/Nipride	Anti-hypertensive, vasodilator Hypertensive crisis	0.5–8 mcg/min
norepinephrine/Levophed	Adrenergic Acute hypotension; shock	8–12 mcg/min; titrate for BP
vasopressin/Pitressin	Vasoconstrictor; sepsis-related hypotension	0.01 units/hour; maximum 0.04 units/hour
Antidysrhythmics		
amiodarone/Cordarone	Antidysrhythmic; VT, SVT A-fib, VF not controlled by first-line medications	Loading: 150 mg over 10 min, then 360 mg over next 6 hours (1 mg/min), then 540 mg over next 18 hours (0.5 mg/min)
diltiazem/Cardizem	Calcium channel blocker; A-fib, A-flutter, PSVT	Bolus: 0.25 mg/kg over 2 min, after 15 min then 0.35 mg/kg; if no response, start infusion 5–15 mg/hr for up to 24 hours
Anticoagulants/Antiplatelets		
abciximab/Reopro	Antiplatelet; glycoprotein IIb/IIIa inhibitor Prevent cardiac ischemia in patients undergoing PCI	Bolus: 0.25 mg/kg given 10–60 min before start of PCI; infuse at 0.125 mcg/kg/min
alteplase/Activase	Thrombolytic enzyme Lysis of obstructing thrombi	Greater than 65 kg: 100 mg total in divided dose of 6–10 mg over 1–2 min; 60 mg over 1 hour; 20 mg over the next hour; 20 mg over the last hour Less than 65 kg: 1.25 mg/kg over 3 hours

(continued)

generic/Trade	Classification and Indication	Dosage
argatroban	Anticoagulant HIT Thrombosis, prophylaxis	2 mcg/kg/min: 50 kg–6 mL/hr 70 kg–8 mL/hr 90 kg–11 mL/hr 110 kg–13 mL/hr 130 kg–16 mL/hr
Bivalirudin/ Angiomax	Anticoagulant; thrombin inhibitor Anticoagulation in conjunction with ASA for unstable angina undergoing PTCA/PCI; co-administer with IIb/IIIa	Bolus: 0.75 mg/kg before procedure, then 1.75 mg/kg/hr during the procedure and up to 4 hours post
eptifibatide/ Integrillin	Antiplatelet; acute coronary syndrome undergoing PCI	ACS: Bolus 180 mcg/kg, then continuous at 2 mcg/kg/min
heparin	Anticoagulant; STEMI in conjunction with fibrinolytics; unstable angina	STEMI: bolus 60 units/kg (4,000 units max); then 12 units/kg/hr infusion Unstable angina: bolus 60 units/kg; then 12 units/kg/hr
tenecteplase/TNKase	Thrombolytic enzyme; AMI	Less than 60 kg: 30 mg over 5 sec Less than 70 kg: 35 mg over 5 sec 70–80 kg: 40 mg over 5 sec 80–90 kg: 45 mg over 5 sec Greater than 90 kg: 50 mg over 5 sec
tirofiban/Aggrastat	Antiplatelet; ACS in combination with heparin	0.4 mcg/kg/min for 30 min; then 0.1 mcg/kg/min for 12–24 hours after angioplasty or arthrectomy

ACS, acute coronary syndrome; A-Fib, atrial fibrillation; A-Flutter, atrial flutter; AMI, acute myocardial infarction; BP, blood pressure; HIT, heparin-induced thrombocytopenia; HTN, hypertension; PCI, percutaneous coronary intervention; PSVT, paroxysmal supraventricular tachycardia; PTCA, percutaneous transluminal coronary angioplasty; STEMI, ST-elevated myocardial infarction; SVT, supraventricular tachycardia; VF, ventricular fibrillation; VT, ventricular tachycardia.

Resources

Burns, S. M., & Delgado, S. A. (2019). *AACN essentials of critical care nursing* (4th ed.). New York, NY: McGraw-Hill.

Diepenbrock, N. H. (2015). *Quick reference to critical care* (5th ed.). Philadelphia, PA: Wolters Kluwer.

Jones, J., & Fix, B. (2015). *Critical care notes: Clinical pocket guide* (2nd ed.). Philadelphia, PA: FA Davis.

Urden, L. D., Stacy, K. M., & Lough, M. E. (2020). *Priorities in critical care nursing* (8th ed.). St. Louis, MO: Elsevier.

Appendix D:
Basic EKG Rhythm Examples

Sinus Rhythm

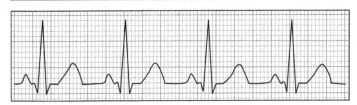

Sinus Bradycardia

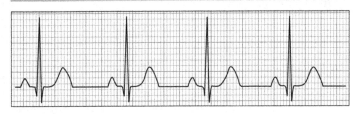

Sinus Tachycardia

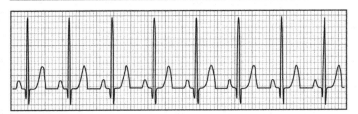

First-Degree Heart Block

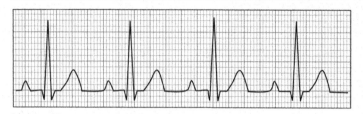

Second-Degree Heart Block, Type I Wenckebach

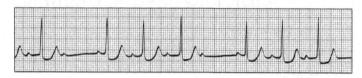

Second-Degree Heart Block, Type II

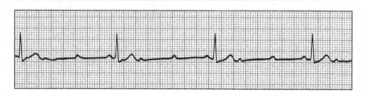

Third-Degree Heart Block

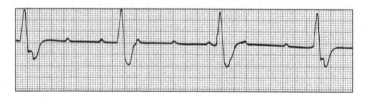

Atrial Flutter

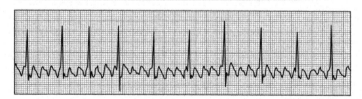

Atrial Fibrillation

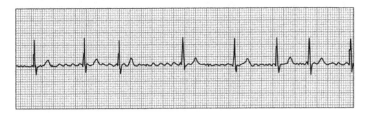

Junctional

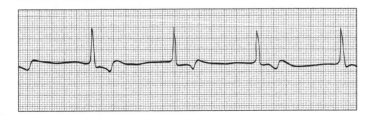

Supraventricular Tachycardia

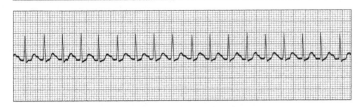

Paroxysmal Supraventricular Tachycardia

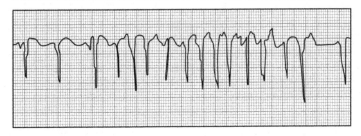

Idioventricular

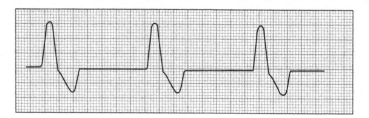

Sinus Rhythm With Unifocal Premature Ventricular Contractions (PVCS)

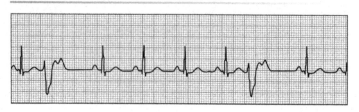

Sinus Rhythm With Multifocal PVCS

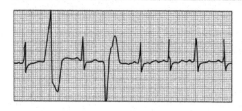

Bigeminal PVCS

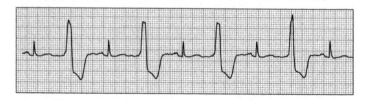

Ventricular Tachycardia

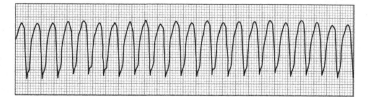

Ventricular Fibrillation

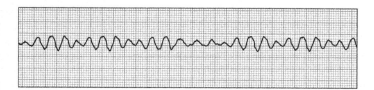

Ventricular Pacing

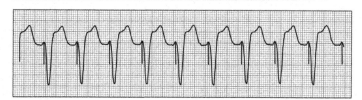

Asystole

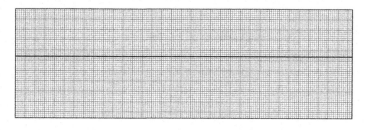

Appendix E: Respiratory and Ventilator Terminology

Assist control (AC): Each time the patient initiates a breath, the ventilator provides a preset tidal volume or preset peak pressure. This mode may also be referred to as intermittent positive pressure ventilation (IPPV).

Controlled mandatory ventilation (CMV): The ventilator controls the frequency of each breath without regard to patient-initiated breaths. Generally used only on unconscious/sedated patients who are pharmacologically paralyzed or who suffered a neurological event where spontaneous respirations are not initiated.

Continuous positive airway pressure (CPAP): Used when weaning the patient from the ventilator. Continuous pressure is maintained throughout inspiration and expiration during spontaneous breathing.

Flow-by ventilation: Used when weaning the patient from the ventilator. A continuous flow of oxygen is through an open circuit. No pressure is supplied to the patient who is breathing spontaneously.

Intermittent mandatory ventilation (IMV): The ventilator is set to deliver a specific number of breaths/minute at a preset tidal volume (TV). If the patient breathes in addition to the preset number of breaths/minute, the ventilator will not deliver a specific TV. May be used as a weaning mode.

Inverse ratio ventilation (I:E): Increases the inspiratory time to provide for increased alveoli filling time, preventing alveoli collapse during rapid expiration. The patient must be sedated and pharmacologically paralyzed. Typically used for patients in acute respiratory distress syndrome (ARDS).

Positive end-expiratory pressure (PEEP): Additional pressure at the end of expiration used to keep alveoli open and promote better oxygen exchange. Use high levels of PEEP cautiously and monitor for barotrauma in the form of pneumothorax, or decreased cardiac output due to increased intrathoracic pressure.

Pressure control (PC): Pressure of the gases delivered is preset and the ventilator delivers each breath to the preset pressure. May be used with I:E.

Pressure support (PS): Used during weaning from mechanical ventilation. When the patient initiates a breath, the ventilator supports the preset pressure level, thus making the flow of gas into the lungs easier.

Synchronized intermittent mandatory ventilation (SIMV): The ventilator is set to deliver a specific number of breaths/minute at a preset tidal volume. If the patient breathes in addition to the preset number of breaths/minute, the ventilator will not deliver a breath at the same time. Generally combined with pressure support and used for weaning.

Volume assured pressure support (VAPS): A combination of volume and pressure control.

Resources

Burns, S. M., & Delgado, S. A. (2019). *AACN essentials of critical care nursing* (4th ed.). New York, NY: McGraw-Hill.

Diepenbrock, N. H. (2015). *Quick reference to critical care* (5th ed.). Philadelphia, PA: Wolters Kluwer.

Jones, J., & Fix, B. (2015). *Critical care notes: Clinical pocket guide* (2nd ed.). Philadelphia, PA: FA Davis.

Urden, L. D., Stacy, K. M., & Lough, M. E. (2020). *Priorities in critical care nursing* (8th ed.). St. Louis, MO: Elsevier.

Appendix F: Acronyms

A:P:	Anteroposterior diameter
AACN:	American Association of Critical-Care Nurses
AANN:	American Association of Neuroscience Nurses
ABG:	Arterial blood gas
ABTC:	American Board of Transplant Certification
AC:	Assist control
ACE:	Angiotensin-converting enzyme
ACLS:	Advanced cardiac life support
ACS:	Acute coronary syndrome
ADH:	Antidiuretic hormone
AKI:	Acute kidney injury
ALF:	Acute lung injury
ANA:	American Nurses Association
ANCC:	American Nurses Credentialing Center
ARDS:	Adult respiratory distress syndrome
ARRA:	American Recovery and Reinvestment Act
ATN:	Acute tubular necrosis
AV:	Arteriovenous
BAI:	Blunt aortic injuries
BIVAD:	Biventricular assist device
BLS:	Basic life support

BP:	blood pressure
BSA:	Body surface area
BUN:	Blood urea nitrogen
CABG:	Coronary artery bypass grafting
CAD:	Coronary artery disease
CAP:	Community acquired pneumonia
CAVH:	Continuous arteriovenous hemofiltration
CAVHD:	Continuous arteriovenous hemodialysis
CCRN:	Critical Care Registered Nurse
CCTN:	Certified Clinical Transplant Nurse
CCU:	Cardiac care unit
CK-MB:	Creatine kinase-muscle/brain
CMC:	Cardiac Medicine Certification
CMV:	Controlled mandatory ventilation
CNRN:	Certified Neuroscience Registered Nurse
CNS:	Central nervous system
CO_2:	Carbon dioxide
COHb:	Carboxyhemoglobin
COPD:	Chronic obstructive pulmonary disease
CPAP:	Continuous positive airway pressure
CPP:	Cerebral perfusion pressure
CPSS:	Cincinnati Prehospital Stroke Scale
CRRT:	Continuous renal replacement therapy
CSC:	Cardiac Surgery Certification
CSF:	Cerebrospinal fluid
CT:	Computed tomography
CVA:	Cerebrovascular accident
CVICU:	Cardiovascular intensive care unit
CVP:	Central venous pressure
CVVH:	Continuous venovenous hemofiltration
CVVHD:	Continuous venovenous hemodialysis
CVVHDF:	Continuous venovenous hemodiafiltration

DBP:	Diastolic blood pressure
DDAVP:	Desmopressin acetate
DI:	Diabetes insipidus
DIC:	Disseminated intravascular coagulation
DKA:	Diabetic ketoacidosis
DVT:	Deep vein thrombosis
ECMO:	Extracorporeal membrane oxygenation
EEG:	Electroencephalogram
EKG:	Electrocardiogram
ELNEC:	End of Life Nursing Education Consortium
EMAR:	Electronic medication administration records
EMR:	Electronic medical record
EOL:	End of life
ETT:	Endotracheal tube
FiO_2:	Fraction of inspired oxygen
GCS:	Glasgow Coma Scale
GFR:	Glomerular filtration rate
GI:	Gastrointestinal
HCO_3:	Bicarbonate
HD:	Hemodialysis
HFJV:	High frequency jet ventilation
HFOV:	High frequency oscillatory ventilation
HFPPV:	High frequency positive pressure ventilation
HFV:	High frequency ventilation
HHS:	Hyperosmolar hyperglycemic state
HITECH:	Health Information Technology for Economic and Clinical Health Act
HVI:	Hollow viscus injury
IABP:	Intra-aortic balloon pump
ICP:	Intracranial pressure
ICU:	Intensive care units
IMV:	Intermittent mandatory ventilation

IPPV:	Intermittent positive pressure ventilation
IPV:	Intimate partner violence
IV:	Intravenous
LBBB:	Left bundle branch block
LGI:	Lower gastrointestinal
LOC:	Level of consciousness
LVAD:	Left ventricular assist devices
MAP:	Mean arterial pressure
MI:	Myocardial infarction
MODS:	Multi-organ dysfunction syndrome
MRA:	Magnetic resonance angiography
MRI:	Magnetic resonance imaging
MVC:	Motor vehicle crash
NeuroICU:	Neurological critical care unit
NG:	Nasogastric tube
NICU:	Neurological intensive care unit
NIHSS:	National Institute of Health Stroke Scale
NPA:	Nurse Practice Act
NSAID:	Nonsteroidal anti-inflammatory drug
NSTEMI:	Non-ST-elevated myocardial infarction
NYHA:	New York Heart Association
PA:	Pulmonary artery
PC:	Pressure control
PCCN:	Progressive Critical Care Nurse
PCI:	Percutaneous coronary intervention
PE:	Pulmonary embolus
PEA:	Pulseless electrical activity
PEEP:	Positive end-expiratory pressure
PET:	Positron emission tomography
PPI:	Proton-pump inhibitor
PS:	Pressure support
PTCA:	Percutaneous transluminal coronary angioplasty

RN:	Registered nurse
rTPA:	Recombinant tissue plasminogen activator
SAH:	Subarachnoid hemorrhage
SBP:	Systolic blood pressure
SCRN:	Stroke Certified Registered Nurse
SCUF:	Slow continuous ultrafiltration
SIADH:	Syndrome of inappropriate secretion of antidiuretic hormone
SICU:	Surgical intensive care unit
SIMV:	Synchronized intermittent mandatory ventilation
SIRS:	Systemic inflammatory response syndrome
SPECT:	Single photo emission tomography
SSC:	Surviving Sepsis Campaign
STEMI:	ST-Elevated myocardial infarction
TBI:	Traumatic brain injury
TCD:	Transcranial Doppler
TeleICU:	Intensive care unit telemedicine
TIA:	Transient ischemic attack
TTT:	Targeted temperature management
TV:	Tidal volume
UGI:	Upper gastrointestinal
USA:	Unstable angina
VAD:	Ventricular assist device
VAP:	Ventilator acquired pneumonia

Index

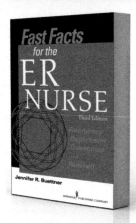
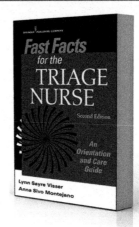
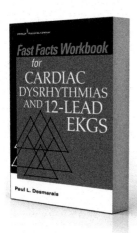
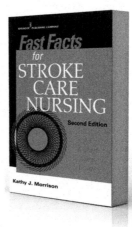